PARENT-LED CBT FOR CHILD ANXIETY

Parent-Led CBT for Child Anxiety

HELPING PARENTS HELP THEIR KIDS

Cathy Creswell
Monika Parkinson
Kerstin Thirlwall
Lucy Willetts

THE GUILFORD PRESS
New York   London

Copyright © 2017 The Guilford Press
A Division of Guilford Publications, Inc.
370 Seventh Avenue, Suite 1200, New York, NY 10001
www.guilford.com

Paperback edition 2019

Printed in the United States of America

This book is printed on acid-free paper.

Last digit is print number: 9   8   7   6   5   4   3   2

The authors have checked with sources believed to be reliable in their efforts to provide information that is complete and generally in accord with the standards of practice that are accepted at the time of publication. However, in view of the possibility of human error or changes in behavioral, mental health, or medical sciences, neither the authors, nor the editor and publisher, nor any other party who has been involved in the preparation or publication of this work warrants that the information contained herein is in every respect accurate or complete, and they are not responsible for any errors or omissions or the results obtained from the use of such information. Readers are encouraged to confirm the information contained in this book with other sources.

Library of Congress Cataloging-in-Publication Data

Names: Creswell, Cathy, author. | Parkinson, Monika, author. | Thirlwall,
    Kerstin, author. | Willetts, Lucy, author.
Title: Parent-led CBT for child anxiety : helping parents help their kids /
    Cathy Creswell, Monika Parkinson, Kerstin Thirlwall, Lucy Willetts.
Description: New York : Guilford Press, [2017] | Includes bibliographical
    references and index.
Identifiers: LCCN 2016031335 | ISBN 9781462527786 (hardcover : alk. paper) |
    ISBN 9781462540808 (paperback: alk. paper)
Subjects: | MESH: Anxiety Disorders—therapy | Child | Child Behavior
    Disorders—therapy | Cognitive Therapy—methods | Parent–Child Relations |
    Patient Education as Topic
Classification: LCC RJ506.A58 | NLM WM 172 | DDC 618.92/8522—dc23
LC record available at https://lccn.loc.gov/2016031335

About the Authors

Cathy Creswell, DClinPsy, PhD, is Professor of Developmental Clinical Psychology in the School of Psychology and Clinical Language Sciences at the University of Reading, United Kingdom. She is also Honorary Consultant Clinical Psychologist and Joint Director of the University of Reading Anxiety and Depression in Young People clinical research unit. Dr. Creswell's research and clinical interests focus on the development and treatment of anxiety disorders in children and adolescents. In addition to numerous academic publications, she is coauthor (with Lucy Willetts) of two self-help books for parents of children with anxiety disorders.

Monika Parkinson, DClinPsy, is a clinical psychologist and Clinical Research Fellow at the University of Reading. She has worked clinically for the U.K. National Health Service and on several large treatment trials at the University of Reading, as well as running her own private practice. Dr. Parkinson's interests focus on identifying effective components of treatments for youth and finding cost-effective ways of supporting families and parents of youth with mental health difficulties. She is coauthor (with Shirley Reynolds) of two self-help books on teenage depression.

Kerstin Thirlwall, DClinPsy, PhD, is a chartered clinical psychologist and Honorary Fellow at the University of Reading. She led a treatment trial funded by the U.K. Medical Research Council that assessed the effectiveness of a guided parent-delivered cognitive-behavioral therapy approach for childhood anxiety disorders. Dr. Thirlwall continues to have a special interest in evidence-based treatments for childhood anxiety disorders, with a particular focus on parent-led approaches; delivers teaching and training to mental health professionals; and provides treatment for children and their families.

Lucy Willetts, DClinPsy, PhD, is a chartered clinical psychologist and accredited cognitive-behavioral therapist. She worked as a clinical psychologist within the U.K. National Health Service for nearly 20 years and most recently was Clinical Director of the Berkshire Child Anxiety Clinic. Dr. Willetts now works in private practice and is Visiting Fellow at the University of Reading. She is coauthor of several books on childhood anxiety.

Acknowledgments

We are extremely grateful to Vanessa Cobham, Xu Fuzhen, Polly Waite, Claire Hill, Brynjar Halldorssen, Debbie Andrews, and Kim Freeman for their feedback on the ideas and early proofs of this book. We would like to particularly thank Liz White for all her help with preparing the manuscript.

Foreword

With more than 150 randomized controlled trials testing treatments for children with anxiety-related problems published as of early 2019, we are lucky to have extensive research literature on treating children with anxiety. In almost two-thirds of those studies, a child-focused cognitive-behavioral or exposure treatment was used as the key intervention. This might suggest that the field is dominated by child-focused treatments and does not involve caregivers in treatment in significant ways. Although this could appear to be true if you look only at how these treatments are described, it is actually a misleading statement in some important ways. And it is exactly those important ways that make the book you are holding so useful and timely. Parents and caregivers are always involved in treatment, but this has rarely been articulated—until the publication of this book.

In reality, child therapy doesn't occur in isolation from parents or caregivers, even when clinicians are working primarily with the child. Caregivers are involved in treatment from the beginning phone call and almost always provide the impetus behind seeking treatment in the first place. In addition, they provide critical assessment information that guides case conceptualization. They bring the child to sessions and assist with home-based assignments. They are the key reporters on how treatment is going. And in many cases, they are critical participants in the change that occurs during treatment. Yet, in many child-focused treatments for anxiety, there is limited guidance for how best to involve and work with caregivers.

Enter this concise, clinically rich guide to how to involve parents in treatment, written by United Kingdom–based authors Cathy Creswell, Monika Parkinson, Kerstin Thirlwall, and Lucy Willetts. Their work focuses on much needed treatments that explicitly involve caregivers. Fortunately for readers, their program not only makes clear how caregivers are involved, the program places the caregiver front and center. As such, they are ahead of the current clinical model, and they have created a volume that guides you through the steps to ensure that parents are involved in a way that promotes reduction in symptoms, if not complete remission.

A number of factors make this book special. First, the book is incredibly practical. There are numerous specific examples showing how to approach tricky situations like encouraging caregivers to buy in to the program and guiding them through the process, while allowing them enough autonomy and providing them with much needed support. With excellent clinical samples, readers are afforded a view into how to put their ideas into action. In addition, model dialogue shows how therapists can phrase some of the more challenging topics.

Second, the book is developmentally sensitive. This is no surprise, really, given the authors' expertise. Still, it is a pleasure to read specific developmental adaptations for a variety of strategies throughout the book. If you are reading this book, you know already that a 6-year-old and a 10-year-old require different approaches. Sadly, not all therapy book authors seem aware of the importance of the vastly different needs of children, even those who are close in age. Readers will be helped by knowing the developmental capacities for change in a given child.

Third, there are focused chapters on some of the most vexing challenges facing therapists working with children who are anxious. For example, there are separate chapters on sleep and school refusal. These two incredibly practical chapters are worth the price of the book. Furthermore, there are three chapters related to helping caregivers who may fit the stereotype of the "helicopter" parent. One chapter focuses on promoting independent problem solving in children, which can be a challenge for hovering parents. We all know how easy it can be to solve a problem for a child in the moment. It saves time. It makes the child happy. Yet, the message the child receives is that when a problem arises, the caregiver will come to the rescue. This is certainly not the approach we are aiming for in most situations.

The authors also cover the important and underappreciated child anxiety strategy of parent modeling. Children are always watching their parents (and others in the environment) for cues on how to handle challenges and fears. The focus on modeling here emphasizes both cognitive and behavioral ways for parents to embrace their role as a model for the child, including how to model a "have a go" attitude.

Lastly and perhaps most importantly, the choice to focus the book on *parent-led* CBT is strong both in its intention and in its execution. I always emphasize to families I work with that my time with them is only 1 hour of the 168 hours in the week. This is only a small percentage of the time that parents spend each week with their children. As therapists, we would need to be highly potent change agents to make a difference in the short period of time we have with clients. The authors have wisely changed the ratio here by involving the caregiver, who will spend much more time with the client. There is excellent material in the book to guide therapists in how to present this idea to caregivers, how to implement it, and how to trouble-shoot when things get tough. And they will get tough.

All in all, the field has been in need of a practical book for therapists looking to involve caregivers deeply in a CBT approach. One need look no further than this excellent book. Turn the page and start reading.

MICHAEL A. SOUTHAM-GEROW, PhD
Virginia Commonwealth University

Contents

Purchasers of this book can download and print the handouts
at *www.guilford.com/creswell-forms* for personal use
or with individual clients (see copyright page for details).

CHAPTER 1

Introduction

Together we have worked with hundreds of parents of children with anxiety disorders, supervised and trained hundreds of clinicians in a range of settings, and conducted research in this area. Our intention in writing this book is to bring together our shared knowledge and experience to guide therapists in working with parents of children with anxiety disorders. All the case studies in the book are based on composites across many cases. The aim of this first chapter is to introduce the background and philosophy of our overall approach. We appreciate that it might be tempting to skip straight to the practical sections, but we encourage you to stick with us so that you have a good understanding of why we do what we do, and ultimately, why we are suggesting that you do the same!

Treatment for Childhood Anxiety Disorders: How Is This Approach Different?

It is now well known that anxiety disorders are among the most common mental health difficulties and that they typically first occur in childhood or adolescence (Kessler et al., 2005). Indeed worldwide prevalence rates suggest that about 6.5% of children are likely to meet diagnostic criteria for an anxiety disorder at any one time (Polanczyk, Salum, Sugaya, Caye, & Rohde, 2015), presenting those children with an increased risk of ongoing anxiety problems as well as other health and social difficulties, most notably, depression (Essau & Gabbidon, 2013).

Both psychological and pharmacological treatments have been evaluated for children with anxiety disorders; however, due to their lower likelihood of side effects, psychological treatments have been recommended as a first line of treatment for preadolescent children (Rynn et al., 2015). The psychological treatments that have been evaluated to date almost all follow a cognitive-behavioral therapy (CBT) approach, which typically involves a therapist working with the child to address anxious thoughts and avoidant behaviors and to develop coping skills. Most of the CBT-based treatments that are available follow, or are based on, the highly influential Coping Cat program, which was developed by Philip Kendall and his colleagues from Temple University, Philadelphia, and was first evaluated in 1994 (Kendall, 1994). There have now been a large number of trials to evaluate these treatments, with, on average, 60% of children being free of their anxiety disorder by the end of treatment (James, James, Cowdrey, Soler, & Choke, 2013). On the whole, the inclusion of parents within or alongside the children's CBT sessions has not been found to improve children's treatment outcomes (e.g., Reynolds, Wilson, Austin, & Hooper, 2012); however, the extent and way in which parents have been involved in treatments have varied substantially across these trials. A more nuanced analysis, in which the extent and manner of parental involvement have been taken into account, has led to the suggestion that actively including parents in treatment, incorporating a specific focus on helping parents reinforce children's brave behaviors (see Chapter 6), and gradually shifting control of the program from the therapist to the parent are associated with significantly better outcomes for children when assessed a year after treatment (with 82% free of their anxiety diagnosis compared to 53–65% following treatments either with limited parental involvement or without an active focus on contingency management and transfer of control; Manassis et al., 2014).

So, we have CBT treatments that work for many children with anxiety disorders, and it appears that involving parents in particular ways can improve children's outcomes over the medium to long term. However, these treatments are often intensive, involving approximately 14–16 hours of face-to-face child–therapist (and parent–therapist) contact, which presents a challenge for many health care systems. Indeed in the United Kingdom it has been suggested that only a quarter of children with a mental health problem will see a mental health professional (Layard, 2008), and of those that do, many do not access practitioners who are suitably trained or confident in delivering CBT (Stallard, Udwin, Goddard, & Hibbert, 2007). It is essential, therefore, that we find ways to deliver treatments efficiently, while making sure that children continue to have good outcomes from treatment. One way in which to do this is to capitalize on the importance of helping parents feel more empowered to deal with their children's difficulties and to *work primarily with parents or carers* (hereafter, "parents") to help them help their children overcome their difficulties with anxiety. In our view, this approach brings many advantages:

- It reduces the burden on children of attending therapy appointments, including missing school and age-appropriate activities and the perceived stigma of attending mental health services.
- It reduces the overall amount of therapy time because
  - There is not the same need for activities and games to increase child engagement and motivation (with working directly with parents, we can often "cut to the chase").
  - Parents can implement CBT strategies within their children's day-to-day life.
- Concerns about longer-term difficulties may make parents more motivated to engage in treatment than children, who may be reluctant to attend.
- Parents are more likely (than therapists) to be present at times when children need to put strategies in place between sessions and help them generalize principles in day-to-day life.
- Parents may be in a better position (than children or therapists) to create opportunities to implement strategies and promote their repetition and generalization between sessions.
- Parents are generally in a better position (than children) to liaise with schools or other agencies to encourage the implementation of useful strategies (while retaining control of this within the family rather than it being taken over by the therapist).
- Treatment provides the opportunity to address any parenting practices that may be inadvertently maintaining child anxiety (see Chapter 2) and, instead, empowers parents to help their children overcome their difficulties.
- Parents can apply the principles and strategies on a familywide basis, potentially helping other children within the family and possibly themselves.
- Parents are more likely (than children) to recall and put strategies in to place if problems recur in the months/years following treatment.
- Parents' lives can be significantly affected by having a child who suffers with anxiety, and treatment provides opportunity for them to gain support.

Parents are the most important agent for change that we can access in helping children to overcome difficulties with anxiety. It is essential that we value parents and help them feel skilled and confident in managing their children's difficulties.

Parent-Led Treatment for Childhood Anxiety Disorders: Does It Work?

As noted above, the majority of treatment trials that have evaluated psychological treatments for children with anxiety disorders have typically involved direct therapeutic work with children, with or without additional input for or from parents. However, in recent years a number of trials have reported positive outcomes for children when the intervention is focused exclusively on parents. This approach was first evaluated in Australia, with the specific aim of supporting families in rural communities who were unable to easily access child mental health services (Rapee, Abbott, & Lyneham, 2006; Lyneham & Rapee, 2006). In these studies, parents of 6- to 12-year-old children were given a book to guide them in how to help their child. Giving the parents the book on its own was associated with a modest impact on children's anxiety problems: 26% of children were free of their anxiety disorder compared to 7% among those who received no treatment. However, the book-based intervention was not as effective as standard group CBT involving children and parents (61% diagnosis free). In a subsequent trial, supplementing the book for parents with therapist support (provided over the telephone) was associated with extremely positive outcomes, with 79% of children being free of their anxiety disorder. Later U.K.-based trials have also demonstrated that children can achieve good outcomes when parent-only treatment is delivered in a group (57% diagnosis free; Cartwright-Hatton et al., 2011) or in a brief format involving only about 5 hours of therapist input (50% diagnosis free; Thirlwall et al., 2013). Of particular note, two trials that have directly compared parent-only treatment to parent and child treatment found no significant differences between treatments in terms of child outcomes, despite the fact that the parent + child treatment involved at least twice the amount of therapist input to deliver parallel parent and child sessions (Waters, Ford, Wharton, & Cobham, 2009; Cobham, 2012; Creswell, Hentges, et al., 2010). Specifically in the Cobham study, a remarkable 95% of children (7–14 years old) were free of all their anxiety disorders after the parents received a brief intervention comprising a 2-hour parent group followed by six phone calls delivered over 2-week intervals to guide the parent through a workbook, compared to 78.3% of children who received a 12-session family-focused CBT treatment and 0% in the wait-list control condition. Although this is still an emerging area for research, it is clear that taking a parent-led approach to treatment can provide an efficient means of bringing about excellent outcomes for children with anxiety disorders.

Guiding parents to put CBT principles into practice in their children's day-to-day life is a brief and effective treatment approach for childhood anxiety disorders.

For Whom Is This Book Intended?

We have written this book for clinicians who work with children with anxiety disorders to provide an overview and a framework for also working with the parents of these children. Although we are assuming a general background in child mental health treatment, we have not assumed any prior knowledge of CBT because we have found that novices in CBT can successfully implement the parent-led treatment approach that we are describing (after brief training and with ongoing supervision; Thirlwall et al., 2013). Furthermore, we have examined the feasibility of this approach within a U.K. primary care mental health service with mental health workers with a broad range of backgrounds (including psychology, social work, nursing and home health visiting) and have found that (again, following brief training and with ongoing supervision) the mental health workers delivered the treatment well and achieved good outcomes (Creswell, Hentges, et al., 2010). However, whether you are a novice or experienced therapist, we strongly recommend that you access regular clinical supervision, which will be essential in supporting the work you do with families.

With Whom Can This Approach Be Used?

Age of the Child

Parent-led approaches to treatment for childhood anxiety disorders have been evaluated with children in ages ranging from 2 years, 7 months (Cartwright-Hatton et al., 2011), up to 14 years (Cobham, 2012), but the majority of study participants have been between 6 or 7 and 12 years of age. Although we have anecdotal reports of the approach being used successfully with both younger and older children (with some adaptations), we do not yet have a firm evidence base on which to recommend the approach, but we would welcome feedback based on your own experiences. Similarly, we have heard anecdotal reports of the approach being used successfully with children with developmental delay and autism spectrum disorders (ASD) (where it might be argued that the increased repetition that comes from working with parents may be particularly useful in promoting generalization;

Puleo & Kendall, 2011); however, as yet we have no solid evidence on which to base recommendations. Finally, the studies of this approach to date have included fairly homogeneous groups in terms of social, economic, cultural, and ethnic backgrounds, and the extent to which the approach is appropriate, acceptable, and effective across, for example, different cultures remains unclear. We would very much welcome any feedback from your experiences of applying the approach in more diverse settings.

Participating Adults

Our preference is to invite the child's primary caregivers in to treatment, so when there is more than one key carer, we encourage them both/all to attend treatment. It may not always be practical for more than one parent to attend every session. Sessions conducted over the telephone may also present challenges when more than one parent is involved, so we ask parents to nominate one of them to be the main point of contact, to commit to attending every session, and to provide feedback to another parent if he or she is not able to join a particular session. If parents are willing, audio recordings of sessions could be shared with a parent who is unable to attend. Of course, it is also sometimes the case that children live with different parents at different times, and that parents do not feel able to come together for their children's treatment. Our view is that the critical factors in deciding who participates in treatment is that (1) the participating parent is able to commit to attending the sessions and (2) is in a position to consistently make relevant changes in their child's life. For example, if a child lives with one parent during the week and another at weekends, and all of the difficulties relate to attending school, it would be critical to have the parent who has to manage those weekday difficulties involved in treatment. The participating parent also needs to be motivated to bring about changes in his or her child's life. For example, from time to time we have worked with families in which one parent is very concerned about the child's anxiety, but the other parent does not share these concerns. As we discuss in Chapter 2, it is obviously important to ascertain each parent's view of the child's difficulties independently, because it is possible that one parent has a particular perception of the other parent's view—for example, that he or she is disinterested or unsupportive—but this may not accurately reflect the other parent's perspective. On the other hand, if it becomes clear that a parent does not consider his or her child to have a problem with anxiety, that parent is unlikely to be motivated to attend therapy sessions focused on helping the child overcome these difficulties. We discuss general considerations for engaging parents and maximizing their motivation throughout the book.

What Does the Treatment Involve?

Fundamental Principles

The overall aim of the treatment is to work collaboratively with parents to help them develop the skills and confidence to support their children in overcoming difficulties with anxiety. In creating an individualized treatment plan, the therapist role is to work with parents to bring together therapist knowledge about the maintenance and treatment of childhood anxiety disorders with the parental knowledge of the child and how that child responds to challenges. Therapists also encourage parents in continuing to work through the program and help them (1) rehearse key skills, (2) recognize their own skills and positive progress, and (3) problem-solve any challenges that might arise. In order for this intervention to be successful, it is critical that parents feel engaged in the treatment process and empowered to make changes in their children's lives.

Content of Sessions

The actual content of the treatment is not dissimilar to other CBT programs for child anxiety disorders, and involves the following elements:

- Establishing clear, achievable treatment goals (Chapter 2).
- Providing psychoeducation and individualizing the treatment model (Chapter 3).
- Promoting independence in day-to-day life (Chapter 4).
- Helping parents promote flexible thinking and a "have a go" attitude (Chapter 5).
- Helping parents support their children in facing their fears (Chapter 6).
- Helping parents promote independent problem solving (Chapter 7).
- Keeping progress going (Chapter 8).

The main differences from other child- and/or parent-focused treatments in terms of the content result from our emphasis on working jointly with parents. For example, to promote parental engagement and empowerment, it is critical that parents have good background information about the treatment program to equip them to identify anxiety appropriately in their children, to feel hopeful about their children's outcomes, to understand the rationale for each element of the treatment program, and to relate these directly to their children's particular difficulties. Because many parents embark on treatment feeling concerned that they have caused their children's difficulties in some way (or that the therapist may think that they have), it is essential that the therapist be explicit about the underlying treatment model and how parents' responses fit in to that. As we discuss further in Chapter 3, although the treatment does set out, when appropriate, to alter parental responses that may inadvertently maintain anxiety, this is not to suggest that parents are to blame. Instead we recognize (1) that parents' responses are largely a response to their children's anxiety, and (2) that highly anxious children may be more susceptible to influence from particular parental responses than their less anxious peers or siblings. Parents may also express concerns that they are not the "right person for the job" of putting CBT principles and strategies in place, for example, because they are not the "expert," or they feel that their child is more likely to "open up" to a therapist. For these reasons, as well as providing clear information about the treatment model, it is also essential that the therapy process encourage parental empowerment from start to finish. Beyond these specific aspects of the content, the strategies used are typically from child-focused CBT approaches, adapted in ways that parents can apply in their day-to-day lives.

One element of treatment that is commonly used in child-focused CBT that we have *not* included is that of relaxation. Often treatment programs involve regular relaxation practice based on the assumption that highly anxious children may have a condition characterized by chronic hyperarousal or that developing relaxation skills will help them manage their arousal at times of challenge. We have not used relaxation within our treatments for a number of years for the following reasons:

- There is no evidence that children with anxiety disorders have "chronic dysregulation" of their physiological arousal (e.g., Alkozei, Cooper, & Creswell, 2014).
- There is evidence that it is important to fully experience elevated anxiety in order to truly face fears and learn to overcome them (e.g., Craske, Treanor, Conway, Zbozinek, & Vervliet, 2014).
- There is recent evidence that the introduction of relaxation is not associated with significant gains in terms of treatment outcomes (Peris et al., 2015).
- We have found that parents and children rarely practice relaxation extensively at home and often find it difficult to do.

Given these factors and the fact that one of the primary advantages of this treatment approach is that it is time-limited and efficient, we have not included relaxation in any of the programs that we have evaluated. Like others (e.g., Rapee, 2000), we have found that this absence does not appear to negatively impact children's outcomes, and families generally report that physiological symptoms subside without a direct focus on relaxation in the treatment.

Structure of Sessions

In order for parents to feel equal (or greater) partners in the treatment with the therapist, it is important that the sessions are predictable in terms of their structure and that parents get the opportunity to contribute to the session agenda. As such, all our sessions adhere to the following structure:

- Agenda setting
- Routine outcome monitoring (Chapter 2) and brief update
- Review of home-based tasks
- Structured session activity
- Consideration of other issues parent adds to agenda
- Confirmation of home-based tasks
- Brief review of session to summarize main elements and to ensure that the parent and therapist have a shared understanding

The Work Happens between Sessions

In order to work efficiently with parents, we typically provide them with written materials to read before and between sessions (e.g., Creswell & Willetts, 2007) so that the therapist–parent contact time can be used in a focused way to recap the material covered, reflect on how the material relates to their child, practice key skills, and problem-solve potential difficulties. As is standard in CBT, the inclusion of home-based tasks is critical because we work on the assumption that it is what happens between sessions, rather than within sessions, that brings about change. To support this approach, we always provide parents with worksheets for guiding activities and recording information. These worksheets also provide a means of reviewing progress in the treatment, and they serve as a resource for parents to refer to in future to help them maintain gains that have been made or to overcome setbacks. We always carefully monitor progress with all home-based tasks, and problem-solve with the parent if he or she had difficulties getting through the material between the sessions. This process clearly emphasizes the importance of the work that parents doing between sessions as well as helping them to overcome any potential obstacles. It is obviously important to explicitly consider any potential difficulties with parents, such as language or literacy obstacles, at the outset and consider pragmatic solutions to these (e.g., involving confederates, making audio recordings of session content).

How the Treatment Is Delivered

Parent-led CBT for childhood anxiety disorders has been evaluated in individual and group formats; however, these two formats have not been directly compared to each other to date. Our view is that there are advantages and disadvantages to either format. A group approach gives parents the opportunity to share their experiences and gain support from other parents potentially experiencing similar challenges (which, in our experience, many parents find invaluable), whereas individual sessions allow for a more specific focus on the individual issues facing particular families. A group approach may not be appealing to all parents, some of whom may feel intimidated or anxious about the format. Certainly dropout rates have been found to be relatively high in some studies that have offered parent-only treatment groups (Waters et al., 2009; Monga, Rosenbloom, Tanha, Owens & Young, 2015), although whether this was due to the group format is not clear. Ultimately, in the absence of clear evidence, decisions on whether to offer group or individual parent-led CBT may depend on factors relating to the context. For example, if the throughput of children with anxiety disorders to the service is fairly low, then it would not be reasonable to keep parents waiting for very long periods while a sufficient group is formed; equally, running a group with a small number of parents may not bring benefits in terms of reducing therapist time. In these circumstances an individual approach would be preferable.

Although we have delivered this parent-led CBT approach in both individual and group formats, here we focus primarily on the individual approach because this is what we have formally evaluated. When this approach has been applied in a group setting, the content covered is typically the same and the main differences relate to considerations involving engaging the group members and managing and making the most of the group format.

Whereas some evaluations of parent-led CBT have been entirely clinic-based, a number of studies have demonstrated good outcomes with a less intensive format of delivery, typically including telephone sessions to support parents in applying principles covered in a workbook or manual (e.g., Lyneham & Rapee, 2006; Thirlwall et al., 2013; Cobham, 2012). Although the approach has been applied entirely remotely to reach rural populations (Lyneham & Rapee, 2006), it has also often been delivered in a combination of face-to-face and telephone support sessions (e.g., Thirlwall et al., 2013; Cobham, 2012). We have found that this "combo" approach offers the opportunity to develop parental motivation and engagement as well as to rehearse key skills in person. As such, most commonly we have delivered parent-led CBT over 8 weekly sessions, but with four of those sessions conducted briefly over the telephone with the primary aim of reviewing progress, problem-solving any difficulties that have arisen, and keeping parents focused on the tasks that fit with that stage of treatment. In our view, having at least weekly contact encourages families to continue to firmly prioritize putting treatment into practice in their busy lives.

Parent-led CBT is a collaborative approach to treatment in which parents are supported in developing skills and confidence to help their children overcome their difficulties with anxiety. Having a clear, consistent structure that emphasizes family work between sessions facilitates collaboration. Individual or group approaches may be beneficial, and much work can be done remotely without bringing parents into the clinic.

How to Use This Book

The chapters that follow are presented in the order that we cover the materials in our sessions, and so the book can be used as a manual following a step-by-step approach. Table 1.1 gives an overview of the content we typically cover in each session to act as a guide for your practice.

TABLE 1.1. Overview of Session Content

Session	Format	Content
1	Face to face	Setting the scene: the treatment model and implications for treatment
2	Face to face	Promoting independence and "have a go" thinking
3	Face to face	Facing fears
4	Telephone	Review
5	Telephone	Review
6	Face to face	Problem solving
7	Telephone	Review
8	Telephone	Review and planning for maintaining progress

We would recommend that you read the whole book before embarking on this treatment, and then revisit each chapter in turn when planning each session. The chapters generally follow a set structure comprising an overview, a brief review of relevant evidence, goals, practical guidance, and consideration of potential sticking points.

We have also included chapters that consider how to apply the approach to specific difficulties that can arise in the context of childhood anxiety disorders or in particularly challenging contexts, specifically:

- Managing sleep difficulties (Chapter 9)
- Managing difficulties with school attendance (Chapter 10)
- Putting the treatment into place in the context of parental mental health difficulties and/or child low mood, behavioral difficulties, and/or social skills difficulties (Chapter 11).

If any of these chapters apply to one of your clients, then you should read the appropriate chapter(s) before embarking on treatment so that the additional material can be incorporated throughout your treatment program. We include some information on assessing and identifying each of these areas in Chapters 2, 9, 10, and 11 to help highlight additional information that may be important to consider in your intervention.

Throughout the book we illustrate the application of particular principles or strategies with case studies and sample scripts based on conversations we have had with parents. These cases and their scripts are not direct representations of encounters we have had, as we are keen to preserve anonymity of the families with which we have worked. Instead we have created examples that bring together elements from different families. There can be a tendency for case examples and scripts to seem contrived when written down. We have tried our best to accurately reflect our experiences and those of the families with which we have worked.

Concluding Words

One of the things that we love about this treatment approach is the sense of empowerment and confidence that we see parents develop. Parents often reflect on the broader benefits this approach has brought to them and their families, and, seeing these alongside the gains children have made is immensely rewarding.

We wish you all the best with applying the principles and strategies in this book and hope that you and the families with which you work will be as excited and enthusiastic about this approach as we have come to be.

CHAPTER 2

Conducting a Comprehensive Assessment and Establishing Treatment Goals

In our experience, a comprehensive assessment is essential to achieve good outcomes from treatment for children and their families. Much of our clinical work with children with anxiety disorders has been conducted in the context of research trials, so we have typically had no choice but to adhere to robust assessments, with a range of standardized measures, and to ensure consistency across all assessments. However, this has been an advantage ultimately because it has shown us how important the assessment information is at the beginning, during, and at the end of treatment. Indeed, evidence exists that using routine outcome measures (ROMs)— that is, measures of symptoms and functioning at the initial assessment and during and at the end of treatment—results in faster improvements in youth with mental health problems (Bickman, Kelley, Breda, de Andrade, & Riemer, 2011). That is not to say that we are recommending that all therapists conduct the exact same assessment as we outline below. Rather it is emphasizing the importance of taking time to collect all the information you need, rather than omitting some because of a sense of urgency or limited resources, because in the long run, a good assessment is likely to lead to a more efficient and effective treatment. In our experience, a comprehensive assessment takes approximately 2–3 hours. We have written this chapter assuming no particular background knowledge, and so we have covered generic clinical skills in addition to more specific, anxiety-focused aspects of the assessment; as such there may be sections that are of less relevance to the experienced clinician.

As we have already said, one of the key aims of parent-led interventions is to empower parents so that they feel competent and confident in supporting their child in overcoming his or her anxieties. As the assessment is typically the first contact with parents, it is important to begin this process of empowerment at this stage. Ensuring that you listen carefully to parents' concerns and the information they offer is crucial, in addition to explicitly letting them know that their observations and opinions are highly valued. Indeed, it is important to reiterate that you will be relying on their feedback and observations throughout the sessions. You should also inquire about what has helped in the past and what they have done that has been beneficial, in order to begin what is a collaborative process, rather than one in which you, as a therapist, have all the answers. By modeling behaviors that you want to see parents use with their children, such as listening to their points of view and encouraging them to speak for themselves, you are empowering parents to take control.

This chapter considers how to structure the assessment, with whom to conduct an assessment, and a range of assessment tools that you can use to assess childhood anxiety disorder and symptoms within the context of parent-led treatment. We also address other issues, such as what to do when communication is limited, and we guide you through postassessment decision making about the applicability of this treatment. Finally, we discuss working collaboratively with parents to set goals for treatment that can be monitored throughout therapy.

Goals of Assessment

Screening

It is important to verify that the child does, in fact, present with some type of anxiety problem before conducting a full clinical assessment, for example, by telephone. This can be done by asking for a brief overview of the child's current difficulties. If there is no evidence of any anxiety-related difficulties and other concerns are paramount, it may not be helpful to conduct a full clinical assessment of anxiety.

Diagnosing Disorders

It is important to identify which specific type(s) of anxiety disorder the child is experiencing in order to target treatment appropriately. Later in this chapter we discuss how to go about doing this by using both structured clinical interviews and questionnaires.

Identifying and Quantifying Symptoms and Behaviors

The combination of a structured clinical interview and questionnaire measures will aid you in identifying and quantifying a child's anxiety symptoms and behaviors, and this information will be useful in formulating and planning the intervention.

Assessing Contextual Factors

A more generic clinical interview, which we outline below, will allow you to assess a range of contextual factors that may be relevant to the child's anxiety difficulties, such as friendship problems, learning issues, and/or stressful life events.

Evaluation and Monitoring Treatment Outcome

A range of questionnaire measures administered at the assessment (and again at various points during the intervention) will allow you to monitor and evaluate treatment outcomes.

Structure of the Assessment

It is important to explain the structure of the assessment to the family at the beginning, including approximate timings for each part, so that both parents and children are aware of exactly what is going to happen. We suggest that you begin the assessment with the whole family together, setting the agenda, including rough timings for each section, and then asking for a brief summary of the child's main difficulties. Make it clear to family members that there will be times for them to talk to you individually during the assessment so that they can raise particular issues then, if they would feel more comfortable. We recommend that you then conduct a structured diagnostic interview separately with the parent(s) and the child. Finally, we recommend that you meet with the parent(s) and the child together again in order to gather information about any contextual factors that might be relevant to the anxiety problem—for example, information about the child's family background, developmental history, and school progress if it is appropriate to discuss these all together (see "Assessment of Contextual Factors" on page 26 for more details; see also Figure 2.1).

It is important to conduct the assessment of anxiety first so that you can ascertain if the child does meet the criteria for an anxiety disorder and thus if this intervention is appropriate. Once you have confirmed an anxiety problem, it is then appropriate to explore possible contextual factors. If you choose to assess contextual factors first, you may find that some of this information is redundant later if the child does not, in fact, have a significant anxiety problem and needs to seek help elsewhere. Similarly, in exploring contextual factors first, you run the risk of placing too much emphasis on these issues; for example, parents may interpret your exploration of the family background and their own anxiety issues as your blaming them for their child's anxiety difficulties.

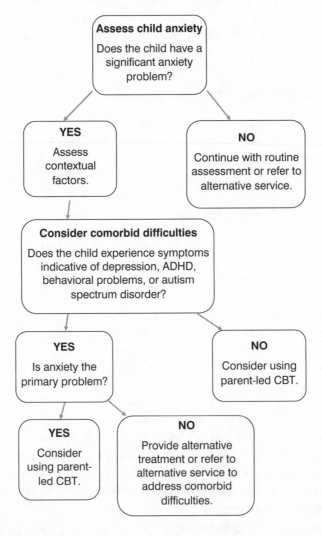

FIGURE 2.1. Deciding whether this is the right treatment for the child.

We would recommend that you gather questionnaire data from the family at the assessment rather than giving them questionnaires to take home. In our experience, you are more likely to elicit complete data if it is all collected as part of the assessment session. The questionnaires can be completed at the beginning, while the family is waiting to be seen, during the assessment (while the parent is participating in the structured clinical interview, and vice versa) or at the end of the assessment.

From Whom to Gather Information

Parent and Child Together

There are advantages to conducting part of the assessment with the parent and child together and, as noted, we would recommend doing so at the beginning of the assessment. Initially, this format allows the child to acclimatize to, and become familiar with, the assessment environment, which is likely to help the child feel more willing to complete part of the assessment alone with the therapist. Another significant advantage of meeting with the parent and child together is the opportunity to directly observe the child's behavior with the parent, and vice versa. For example, some children may cling to their parent and expect the parent to speak for them; this type of response provides useful information both about the child's level of anxiety and about the ways in which the parent may respond to the child.

We would initially ask the child if he or she would like to tell us about his or her difficulties. If the child prefers that the parent speak first, we would then check with the child periodically if the parent has "got it right" and if there is anything else the child would like to add or say. At this stage, listening carefully to both parent and child, as well as displaying empathy and acknowledging any distress, is crucial to fostering engagement.

Parents

In our experience, it is important to create an opportunity to speak to the parent separately from the child. In this age group, children will sometimes express their anxiety to their parents. Parents are thus able to comment on their children's thoughts and worries and any physiological symptoms of anxiety. There are also areas in which parents bring particular expertise to the assessment process. For example, parents are likely to be able to give excellent information about how their children behave when they are anxious, whereas children may be more reluctant to tell therapists what they are currently avoiding. This might be the case particularly for children who experience social anxiety, and are perhaps eager to please or to present themselves well or as the same as their peers. In addition, parents are usually in a better position than their children to reflect on how their children's anxiety interferes with the children and family's everyday life. Similarly, they may be more reliable informants of historical information such as the onset of the problem, its course over time, particular triggers, and influential events. Parents also tend to be more reliable informants than children when it comes to assessing behavioral difficulties (Jensen et al., 1999), and it has certainly been found that parents report more externalizing problems than do children (Silverman & Nelles, 1988).

Parents' reports about their children's anxiety are inevitably influenced by their own values, views, and experiences. For one parent, a behavior or its absence might be seen as normal or at least acceptable, whereas for another, it may be seen as a significant problem (e.g., a child sleeping in a parent's bed). The same may apply to an anxious thought or worry. For example, one parent may feel that it is normal for a child to be worried about being taken by a stranger, whereas another may feel it is irrational and unhelpful. The parent's own anxious thoughts and behaviors will inevitably affect how the parent views his or her child's anxiety. A parent who experiences similar anxieties may be more alert to the child's anxieties or perhaps more accepting of them. Indeed, Briggs-Gowan, Carter, and Schwab-Stone (1996) found that there was a significant correlation between maternal anxiety and depression and a mother's report of her child's anxiety. The researchers concluded that some level of projection or misinterpretation may partly explain these findings, but they also observed that anxious or depressed mothers may have a lower threshold for identifying behaviors as problematic that would typically be considered as age-appropriate. It is thus important to be mindful of a parent's own anxieties and how these might impact on his or her view of the child's anxiety. For this and other reasons, it is also important to gather information from both parents when possible; later in the chapter we address the issue of how to include noncustodial parents in the "Noncustodial Parents" section on page 32.

The Child

Although parents are generally excellent informants regarding the difficulties their children are having with anxiety, it is also crucial to gather information from the children themselves for several reasons. First, anxious thoughts and worries are an internal process best described by each child. Second, some children may have avoided talking to their parents about their anxiety for fear of upsetting them or not being taken seriously.

Third, some parents may misunderstand or have a different perspective on exactly what their children are anxious about and how it interferes in their everyday lives, Fourth, there may be things that parents have either missed/overlooked or dismissed as unimportant, which may be important. Children are usually well able to describe what they are thinking from about the age of 8. All in all, a thorough assessment of the child can help ensure that the clinician accurately understands the nature of the child's anxious thoughts.

• **What do I do if the child is not able to separate from the parent?** Some children find it hard to participate in an assessment separately from their parent, particularly those with significant separation or social anxiety. In order to make the process easier, we let the child know where the parent will be while we are talking to him or her separately and assure the child that he or she can ask to see the parent at any point. It is important to convey confidence in the child's ability to manage this situation and to provide the parent with clear direction regarding what to do. If the child still struggles to separate from the parent, we may conduct this part of assessment in the same room as the parent, but as physically far away as possible. We may also negotiate with the child to be separated for 5 minutes only to begin with, which in practice often leads to the child's being able to tolerate separation for longer periods of time. Alternatively, we talk to the child with the parent in situ, but ask the parent to allow the child to respond to questions, ideally without assistance or interruption.

• **What do I do if the child refuses to attend the assessment?** Some children are so anxious that they refuse to attend the assessment. Similarly, some parents are concerned that due to their children's high level of anxiety, attending an assessment will be too difficult or traumatic for them. We recommend that you actively encourage the parent to bring the child to the assessment. In advance of the assessment, it is helpful to explain clearly to the parent exactly what the assessment will entail so that both parent and child know what to expect; this in itself is sometimes enough to reduce the child's anxiety and to enable him or her to feel comfortable enough to attend the appointment. It is also beneficial to normalize the child's feelings about attending and to let the parent know that, on the whole, children who do participate in this type of assessment find it manageable and often helpful. Children often comment that they "feel better" after the assessment, and they relate this improved feeling to being able to talk about their problems and hearing that other children experience very similar anxieties.

If, after having shared the above information with the parent, he or she still reports that the child is refusing to attend, it would be worthwhile to consider using a graded approach to the assessment. For example, the child could attend the assessment but does not have to talk; or the child could come with the parent but wait in the waiting room and simply fill in the questionnaires; or, if the service setting allows, the child could be seen in the home or another setting where he or she feels more comfortable.

If the parent is not able or willing to bring the child to the assessment, we would recommend that you meet with the parent alone and conduct as much of the assessment as you are able without the child present. At this time, you can also problem-solve with the parent about how to enable the child to come to a future session so that you could complete your assessment.

Other Informants

Children spend much of their time in school and thus other obvious informants regarding their anxiety difficulties are teachers or other key school staff. Children in primary school tend to have one teacher who knows the child very well and thus can provide useful information about the child's anxiety levels, how the anxiety presents, and how it potentially interferes with school. Some children's anxiety difficulties do not interfere within school; for example, a child whose fears are specific to sleeping alone. However, for many children, anxiety disorders do present difficulties, at least part of the time, in school. In our clinical experience, children with separation anxiety, social anxiety, agoraphobia, or other phobias, as well as those with generalized anxiety, often report high levels of anxiety at the beginning of or during the school day.

In our view, it is helpful to have a perspective from the school regarding the child's anxiety, although this is not essential if the child and parent do not report any interference in the school setting. However, there are particular circumstances where it is really important to talk to the child's teacher, and at these times it will be crucial to explain why to the parent. You will, of course, need parental consent to talk to school personnel, so you will need to present a clear rationale to the parent for this action. Circumstances in which we would deem a school perspective essential are:

- School refusal
- Anxiety about (or problems with) peer relations
- Social skills difficulties
- Anxiety about academic performance
- Bullying

Types of Assessment Tools

Structured Clinical Interviews for Childhood Anxiety

We would recommend using a structured clinical interview to assess anxiety disorders in order to gather comprehensive information about the child's anxiety difficulties. Bearing in mind that most children present with a number of comorbid anxiety disorders (Waite & Creswell, 2014), it is important to ask questions about a range of anxiety conditions, not just the presenting difficulty.

There are several structured clinical interviews that have been developed for use with children. The most commonly used interview to assess anxiety and common comorbid conditions (including behavior and mood disorders, as well as screening questions relating to, e.g., eating disorders and psychosis) is the Anxiety Disorders Interview Schedule for Children (ADIS-IV: C/P; Silverman & Albano, 1996). The anxiety sections of this interview systematically explore the number and types of symptoms that are experienced in relation to each disorder, in addition to the degree to which symptoms are associated with avoidance or distress, and the extent of interference caused. This structure allows you to ascertain if the child meets the criteria for an anxiety disorder (DSM-IV) and to assign a clinical severity rating (CSR). Thus the ADIS-IV: C/P allows you to ascertain what the primary problem is at the start of treatment (and potentially what the initial focus of treatment should be) and also provides a useful measurement of change over time. The instrument has a proforma for both parents and children that should be administered separately. The standard administration of the ADIS-IV: C/P allocates a diagnosis if the child meets criteria on the basis of either the child or the parent's report and the higher of the two CSRs is allocated. The ADIS IV: C/P has satisfactory to excellent test–retest reliability (Silverman, Saavedra, & Pina, 2001) and interrater agreement (Lyneham, Abbott & Rapee, 2007). Becoming familiar with a structured assessment such as the ADIS is very worthwhile because it provides an excellent grounding for understanding the presentation of anxiety disorders in children and how to assess these thoroughly. The ADIS-IV: C/P is available to purchase online. It is recommended that clinicians receive training prior to using it in a clinical or research setting.

If you are unable to access a structured clinical interview, the DSM-5 (American Psychiatric Association, 2013) criteria can be used to guide your assessment of anxiety. These provide a clear description of symptoms, avoidance, and level of interference required for a child to meet the diagnostic criteria for a particular anxiety disorder.

Symptom Questionnaires

A wide range of questionnaires that have been designed to measure anxiety symptoms in children, and we outline some of the most commonly used measures in this section. There is often a temptation to use multiple measures, but doing so can be burdensome to the family, so it is important to think carefully about what information you need and how you are going to use it when selecting a questionnaire. For example, questionnaires can provide information to support the conclusions you draw from your clinical interview (i.e., in terms of identifying particular areas of difficulty with anxiety and comorbid difficulties), and can also be used as a measure of symptom change throughout treatment. Some questionnaires have subscales that focus on symptoms associated with a particular anxiety disorder, which is often a useful way of measuring symptoms of a particular disorder on a session-by-session basis without significantly increasing the burden you place on the child and family. As with clinical interviews, questionnaire data should be gathered from both the child and parent whenever possible. However, with this age group it may be necessary to help children read items and to check their understanding to ensure that their report is valid. As this program is designed as a generic anxiety intervention (i.e., you can use it to address a range of different anxiety problems), we focus on questionnaires that provide information about a range of anxiety difficulties, rather than on disorder-specific questionnaires.

Here we outline three widely used generic anxiety questionnaires for children. The Spence Children's Anxiety Scale (SCAS) and the Revised Child Anxiety and Depression Scale (RCADS) both include a separate parent and child report version, whereas the Multidimensional Anxiety Scale for Children (MASC) only has a self-report version for children. All three questionnaires include subscales that differ slightly between questionnaires. The subscales on the SCAS and RCADS correspond directly to diagnostic categories of anxiety. Of note, the RCADS also includes a measure of depression, which can be helpful in assessing comorbid low mood. The SCAS, RCADS, and MASC are not available in a teacher report form, so we also describe the School Anxiety Scale—Teacher Report (SAS-TR), which can be helpful to establish whether anxiety is a significant issue in school.

Spence Children's Anxiety Scale

The SCAS (Spence, 1998) is a 44-item questionnaire with a child, parent, and preschool version (Nauta et al., 2004; Spence, Rapee, McDonald, &

Ingram, 2001). The SCAS measures subtypes of anxiety difficulties, in line with diagnostic categories, and provides both a total anxiety score and subscale scores. It covers the following areas: separation anxiety, social phobia, obsessive–compulsive disorder (OCD), panic/agoraphobia, physical injury fears, and generalized anxiety. The questionnaire is available online free of charge (*www.scaswebsite.com*), as are normative data and standardized scores for children ages 8–15 years. Both parent and child versions of the questionnaire demonstrate satisfactory to excellent reliability and have been found to differentiate between anxious and nonanxious children (Muris, Merckelbach, Ollendick, King, & Bogie, 2002; Spence, 1998).

Revised Children's Anxiety and Depression Scale

The RCADS (Chorpita, Yim, Moffitt, Umemoto, & Francis, 2000) is a 47-item questionnaire with both a child and parent report version. This questionnaire was developed from the SCAS questionnaire. The physical injury scale has been omitted, due to low internal consistency, and some changes were made to the generalized anxiety disorder (GAD) subscale. A measure of depression was also added. The RCADS measures six areas of concern: separation anxiety, social phobia, panic, GAD, OCD, and depression. Age-related norms are available for children ages 6–18 years. The questionnaire is available online free of change (*www.childfirst.ucla.edu/resources.html*) and an Excel spreadsheet that calculates subscale and total scores, plots the data, and provides standardized scores is also available online at no cost. A total anxiety score and a total anxiety and depression (internalizing) score are provided. The RCADS shows acceptable internal consistency and good convergent validity and test–retest reliability (de Ross, Gullone, & Chorpita, 2002; Chorpita et al., 2000). The RCADS has also demonstrated the ability to discriminate between anxiety and depressive disorders and between the targeted anxiety disorders (Ebesutani et al., 2010). This instrument has been incorporated into the portfolio of pre- and post- and session-by-session measures used nationally by the Children and Young People's Project (CYP) Improving Access to Psychological Therapies (IAPT; CYP IAPT; *www.cypiapt.org*) and is thus widely used in the United Kingdom.

Multidimensional Anxiety Scale for Children, Second Edition (MASC-2)

The MASC-2 (March, 2012) is a 50-item self- and parent-report measure of anxiety and has six scales: GAD index, social anxiety, separation anxiety/phobias, physical symptoms, harm avoidance, and obsessions and compulsions. It has strong internal consistency, excellent test–retest reliability, and good discriminative validity (March, 2012). At the time of publication of this book, MASC-2 was available to purchase online (*www.mhs.com*).

School Anxiety Scale—Teacher Report

The SAS-TR (Lyneham, Street, Abbott, & Rapee, 2008) is a 16-item questionnaire designed to assess child anxiety via teacher report. It has two subscales: social anxiety and generalized anxiety. It has been developed for use with 5- to 12-year-old children. The SAS-TR has demonstrated acceptable internal consistency and correlates with parent reports of child anxiety. It has also been shown to discriminate between clinical and community groups and to be sensitive to change following treatment (Lyneham et al., 2008). The SAS-TR is available online free of charge (*www.centreforemotionalhealth.com.au*).

Measures of the Impact of Child Anxiety

In order to monitor treatment gains, it can be useful to include a clinician checklist or questionnaire that measures the *impact* of the child's anxiety difficulties on various aspects of his or her life, including school and education, friendships, and home life, such as those described in the following sections.

Pediatric Anxiety Rating Scale

The Pediatric Anxiety Rating Scale (PARS; Research Units on Pediatric Psychopharmacology Anxiety Study Group, 2002) is administered by clinicians as an interview to both the parent and child together. It measures symptom severity and impairment in relation to three types of anxiety disorder (GAD, separation anxiety disorder, and social phobia). It comprises 50 items regarding anxiety and seven global items. The PARS has been administered to children ages 7–17 years and has been found to have acceptable reliability and validity (Research Units on Pediatric Psychopharmacology Anxiety Study Group, 2002), and there is good evidence that it is sensitive to change in both CBT interventions and those involving medication (Caporino et al., 2013). At the time of publication, this instrument was available online free of charge (*www.sciencedirect.com/science/article/pii/S0890856709609552*).

Child Anxiety Impact Scale

The Child Anxiety Impact Scale (CAIS; Langley, Bergman, McCracken, & Piacentini, 2004) is a questionnaire that measures the impact of anxiety on a child's psychosocial functioning and includes areas of functioning related to school, home, and friends. It has both a parent and child version, which each have 33 items; these include items about interference in specific areas of life in addition to items measuring overall interference in each of the three areas of functioning (Langley et al., 2004). It has been administered to children ages 7–17 years and has shown to have good reliability and validity (Langley et al., 2013) and also to be sensitive to diagnostic change (Evans, Thirlwall, Cooper, & Creswell, in press).

Child Anxiety Life Interference Scale

The Child Anxiety Life Interference Scale (CALIS; Lyneham et al., 2013) measures the level of interference a child's anxiety causes in both his or her life and the parents' lives and includes the following domains: home, school, social life, and activities. It is a much shorter questionnaire than the CAIS and includes a general question about the child's anxiety and distress and then a series of questions about his or her functioning (eight items). The parent report also includes a series of seven items specifically about the impact the child's anxiety has on the parent's life (e.g., the parent's relationship with his or her partner or with friends). The CALIS has demonstrated acceptable to excellent validity and reliability and is able to distinguish between anxious and nonanxious groups. It is also sensitive to change following psychological treatment (Lyneham et al., 2013). This questionnaire is available online free of charge (*www.centreforemotionalhealth.com.au*).

Behavioral Avoidance Tasks

There are a number of limitations to parent and child reports (both interviews and questionnaires) in assessing a child's difficulties with anxiety. Children (and/or parents) report only what they are willing and able to report (e.g., Nisbett & Wilson, 1977). As a result, answers may be biased by social desirability, a child's limited ability to be introspective, and experimenter demands (e.g., Bijttebier, Vasey, & Braet, 2003). The use of a direct observation of anxiety is likely to overcome some of these difficulties.

Behavioral avoidance tasks (BATS) have been most commonly used in relation to specific phobias. However, they have also been used in relation to OCD and have been found to have good convergent and divergent validity within this context and are sensitive to the effects of treatment (Steketee, Frost, & Bogart, 1996). BATS usually involve the child's exposure to a feared stimulus (e.g., a spider). The child is typically asked to engage is a series of graded stimulus-related tasks. A key advantage to this type of assessment is that it provides highly reliable data about the extent and severity of the child's avoidance of a particular stimulus. It is easiest to design and implement for specific phobias when there are very clear and well-defined stimuli that are avoided. Excellent test–retest reliability has been demonstrated for BATS (e.g., Hamilton & King, 1991).

BATS require a certain amount of time and planning in order to tailor the task to a child's particular anxiety difficulty. However, they provide invaluable information, as noted above, about a variety of anxiety-related components and can also provide useful information about parental responses to the child's anxiety.

Assessment of Contextual Factors

In addition to a diagnostic interview, it is important to have a good understanding of the child's developmental history, family background, and schooling. Eliciting this information helps you to (1) rule out developmental disorders that may be contributing to an anxiety problem and/or (2) ascertain if the child is experiencing academic or social problems at school or (3) if there is a particular disturbance within the family that may be contributing to his or her high levels of anxiety and that may need to be addressed. Following is a list of questions that we suggest you ask to elicit this information:

"Were there any difficulties during pregnancy or the child's birth?"

"Did the child reach his or her developmental milestones at an appropriate age?"

"Did the child experience any difficulties with sleeping, eating or socializing as a toddler and young child?"

"Has the child had any significant health problems?"

"Did the child experience any difficulties (anxiety, social, or behavioral) on starting nursery school, preschool, or school?"

"How is the child progressing at school currently?"

"Has the child experienced any significant difficulties with learning, social interaction (including bullying), or behavior since starting school?"

"Has the child experienced any significant life events during his or her lifetime (e.g., bereavement, significant transition such as relocating or changing schools, significant ill health of family member, divorce of parents)?"

"Who lives at home with the child?"

"Are there any current stresses within the family?"

"Have there been any significant changes in family composition?"

"Has anyone else in the family experienced significant anxiety or any other psychological difficulties (e.g., depression, behavioral difficulties) either currently or in the past (or as a child)?"

"If so, has that person undergone any intervention for his or her difficulties?"

The last two questions clearly need to be raised in a sensitive way as the parent may well feel that he or she is being blamed for the child's difficulties. We would suggest introducing these questions in the following way:

"Anxiety and other psychological difficulties often run in families, and it is therefore helpful for us to know if there is any family history of these types of problems.

"Although people often worry that they are somehow to blame, it can sometimes be advantageous if another family member has experienced anxiety and/or has accessed support or overcome difficulties independently as they will then be in a good position to help the child in doing the same."

It can be helpful to explore how parents currently respond toward their children when they are anxious. However, given the sensitivity associated with asking these questions and the likelihood that parents may interpret this line of questioning as blaming, we do not ask about this area in the initial assessment. Instead we explore the area gently with parents once treatment is under way, when the relationship with the therapist has developed, and when there is the scope to discuss it more thoroughly (see Chapters 3 and 4).

Assessment of Barriers to Treatment

It is also important to assess whether parents are going to be able to access this particular intervention. It is essential to consider if the parents' literacy levels, availability to attend sessions, motivation to support the child in overcoming anxieties, and any other issues may be a barrier to delivering this type of intervention. The questions we might ask to explore these issues include the following:

> "Some parents struggle to read material between sessions, sometimes because they are not comfortable with reading, and it is really helpful for us to know if this is likely to be a problem in advance. Do you think this might be an issue for you?"

> "In our experience, regular attendance at sessions is essential. When parents have not been able to attend regular appointments, we have made much less progress in helping their child overcome difficulties with anxiety. Will you be able to commit to weekly sessions? Is there anything that might get in the way of this?"

> "It is hard work helping a child to overcome [his or her] anxieties, and it requires a certain amount of effort on the part of the parent. I will help you through this, but it is important to choose a time to engage in these sessions when you can dedicate time and energy to working with your child on these difficulties. Do you think you can do this at the moment?"

> "Is there anything else that you think might get in the way of us working together to help your child overcome his or her difficulties?"

Considering Comorbid Problems

Depression

Although depression is not highly comorbid with anxiety disorders in this age group (only 1% of children at this age meet the diagnosis for depression; Waite & Creswell, 2014), some degree of low mood is commonly secondary to severe anxiety difficulties, and if present, may impact on the success of your intervention.

Anxiety disorder diagnostic interviews include sections on the assessment of low mood; for example, the ADIS-IV: C/P includes assessments of both major depressive disorder and dysthymia, the latter being a pervasive mood disorder that affects the child's mood more than 50% of the time. Similarly, the RCADS includes a subsection assessing symptoms of depression. We would recommend that you use both types of assessment tools; the use of a structured clinical interview ensures the collection of comprehensive information about low mood and allows you to decide if the child meets diagnostic criteria for depression, and the use of a standardized questionnaire allows you to monitor and compare symptoms and severity at the initial assessment to other points during and at the end of the intervention. (See Chapter 11 for more information on working with anxiety in the context of comorbid difficulties such as depression.)

Although it is less common with the younger age group we focus on here than older children, even young children with comorbid depression may verbalize the desire to harm themselves and can experience suicidal ideation. It is crucial that a full risk assessment is conducted if this is the case and appropriate action taken to initially ensure that the child is safe and that he or she then receives support and appropriate intervention.

Attention-Deficit/Hyperactivity Disorder

Anxiety disorder in childhood can coexist with attention-deficit/hyperactivity disorder (ADHD), with 6% of children with an anxiety disorder experiencing attention-deficit difficulties (Waite & Creswell, 2014). Once again, the ADIS-IV: C/P includes a section assessing for ADHD, although you will need to seek a more specialist assessment in order to ascertain if the child fully meets the criteria for this particular difficulty. One assessment tool that is commonly used to screen for ADHD is the Strengths and Difficulties Questionnaire (SDQ; Goodman, 1997), which is available online free of charge (*www.sdqinfo.com*). (For further information about working with anxiety in the context of comorbid difficulties such as ADHD, see Chapter 11.)

Oppositional Defiant Disorder/Conduct Disorder

Anxiety disorders and behavioral difficulties also coexist, with up to 6% children with anxiety difficulties also exhibiting oppositional defiant disorder (ODD; Waite & Creswell, 2014). The ADIS-IV: C/P includes a section that measures ODD and conduct disorder (CD). ODD and CD can also be identified using screening tools such as the SDQ (Goodman, 1997), which, as noted above, is available online free of charge (*www.sdqinfo.com*). However, in order to gather more robust diagnostic information, a specialist assessment is recommended. (See Chapter 11 for more information on working with anxiety in the context of comorbid difficulties such as behavioral difficulties.)

Autism Spectrum Disorder

Anxiety disorders are common in children with autism spectrum disorder (ASD); as many as 84% of children with ASD meet diagnostic criteria for an anxiety disorder (Muris, Steerneman, Merkelbach, Holdrinet, & Meesters, 1998). As noted in Chapter 1, the strategies described in this book have not been evaluated for use with children with anxiety problems who also meet the criteria for ASD, and a different approach may need to be considered in this context.

There are a number of screening questionnaires that can be used to monitor a possible ASD diagnosis, including the Children's Communication Checklist (CCC-2; Bishop, 2003) and the Social Communication Questionnaire (SCQ; Rutter, Bailey, & Lord, 2003). The former is suitable for both parent and teacher report, whereas the SCQ is designed for primary caregivers. Both are available for purchase online (*www.pearsonclinical.co.uk*; *www.hogrefe.co.uk*). However, ultimately, it is recommended that you refer to a specialist service if you are concerned that the child may have some characteristics of an ASD for a full assessment of his or her needs.

Treating Anxiety within the Context of Comorbid Difficulties

It is perfectly possible to focus on and treat anxiety difficulties in the context of the above disorders. However, in order to decide whether to (1) provide an alternative treatment, (2) refer the child to a specialist service for treatment of the comorbid difficulty, or (3) treat the anxiety disorder in the first instance, we recommend that you consider the following issues:

- What is the primary problem?
- Are the symptoms of the comorbid disorder a barrier to implementing this intervention?
- Will the child be able to engage in the strategies outlined in this book with his or her parent, despite these difficulties?
- Are the child's symptoms of the comorbid disorder contributing to his or her anxiety levels; for example, is the child anxious about not doing well enough in schoolwork because he or she is not able to concentrate?

In our experience, symptoms or behaviors associated with other disorders (e.g., attentional difficulties, low mood) sometimes improve as a child's anxiety level reduces during treatment. For this reason, it is important to monitor these difficulties in order to make a decision regarding the need for further input for the comorbid difficulties at the end of treatment. In the case of a child with ASD, it is important to consider the impact of the social communication difficulties on his or her ability to access this type of CBT intervention, and adjustments may need to be made to the program in order for it to be accessible to the child. (For further discussion about comorbid mood disorders and behavior difficulties, see Chapter 11.)

Other Considerations

Age of the Child

There is a need to be cautious when assessing younger children to ensure that the information you collect is reliable. In our experience, children ages 8 years and over, with age-appropriate development, are generally able to participate in a structured clinical interview and complete an anxiety questionnaire; our experience is borne out by the age guidance for these measures. For younger children, questions may need to be simplified and scales may need to be reduced to a simpler format (e.g., to a 3-point scale). More weight should be given to parental report, and in some cases, you will need to rely wholly on parental report to make a clinical judgment about diagnosis, although the child's comments can inform your overall assessment.

Communication Issues

Many children who experience difficulties with anxiety, particularly those with high levels of social anxiety and those with selective mutism, may find it very difficult to talk to a stranger, and thus the context of the assessment may bring particular challenges for them. A few simple strategies may help:

Introduction
- Emphasize that there are no right or wrong answers.
- Use developmentally appropriate language—keep it simple.
- Normalize and acknowledge the child's difficulties in speaking to an unfamiliar adult.

Questionnaires
- Start with standardized questionnaires; a nonverbal task with a shared focus of attention away from the child can help, and it also serves to normalize anxiety.
- Once again, emphasize that there are no right or wrong answers.

Clinical Interview

- Talk about nonproblematic areas first, using visual materials as a shared focus of attention (e.g., draw a family tree, talk about hobbies).
- If the child is unable to respond verbally, use questions that require a yes or no answer initially and build up to open questions.
- If the child is unable to respond with a yes or no, negotiate a nod or shake of the head as a response or a written answer if preferred.
- Rate anxiety by pointing to an anxiety scale (e.g., ADIS-IV: P/C thermometer or a scale representing emotional faces).
- Use pictures of particular anxiety subtypes or fears and ask the child to circle ones that are relevant to him or her (e.g., Cool Kids Program; Rapee, Lyneham, et al., 2006).

Noncustodial Parents

As noted in Chapter 1, it is crucial that the parent who is ultimately able to attend all treatment sessions and consistently make relevant changes in the child's life is the parent who becomes involved in treatment and thus is present for the assessment. If there is more than one parent, but both parents are not able to attend the assessment, it will still be important to ask the parent who is not attending the appointment with the child to provide information to inform the assessment wherever possible. When parents are separated, it can be more difficult gaining information from both of them. Some separated parents are happy to attend together; however, for those who are not, we would either conduct a second assessment with the nonattending parent by telephone or invite him or her into the clinic for a separate session. If both parents do not have parental responsibility for the child, consent will need to be gained from the parent who has parental responsibility before talking to the other parent. When there is disagreement between parents about whom should be involved, we would recommend seeking legal advice from your service or professional body to ensure that you are following the correct procedure.

It is not uncommon for separated parents to give very different accounts of the child's anxiety difficulties. This is most commonly due to the varied expressions of anxiety by the child in the two different settings. We have worked with families in which the noncustodial parent has felt strongly that the higher reported anxiety levels are a symptom of the custodial parent's own anxiety. Although this is possible, it is often not the case, but may be explained by one or more of a number of factors:

- The child is more comfortable in expressing his or her anxiety with the custodial parent.
- The child has to face more anxiety-provoking situations in the care of his or her custodial parent (e.g., school, playing with friends).
- There are more fun and/or non-anxiety-provoking activities scheduled during the noncustodial parent's contact.
- The child conceals his or her anxiety from the noncustodial parent.

It is thus important to objectively analyze the information you have collected and try to make sense of discrepancies in reporting, while modeling a nonblaming approach to making sense of the child's anxiety difficulties.

How to Decide on the Most Appropriate Course of Action

Having completed your assessment, you will need to decide on the most appropriate course of action for the child and family. By considering the questions that follow, we hope that you will be able to make an informed decision about whether to use this intervention with the family or whether an alternative course of action is required.

Does the Child Meet the Criteria for an Anxiety Disorder?

CBT is the recommended treatment approach for childhood anxiety disorders and has a robust evidence base (James, Soler, & Weatherall, 2005). Thus if the child does meet the criteria for an anxiety disorder, CBT should be the treatment offered to the family. Of course, CBT can be delivered individually to the child or via the parents, but working via the parents may be a more efficient approach.

Is the Child's Anxiety Difficulty the Primary Problem?

Where there is a distinct and discrete anxiety problem, it may be possible to tackle it using this program in the presence of other difficulties (Thirlwall, Cooper, & Creswell, 2016) as long as the anxiety problem is not a response to, or being maintained by, another difficulty. (See Chapter 11 for more information on working with anxiety in the context of comorbid difficulties.)

Does the Child Show Signs of an ASD or Other Developmental Disorder or Problem?

Currently, there is no evidence base for the efficacy of this sort of parent-led intervention that we describe here for children with anxiety difficulties and ASD. However, from our clinical experience and that of our colleagues, we would conclude that this approach may well be helpful for use with children with ASD. However, adaptions will need to be made to take account of the child's specific difficulties. Indeed, there is an emerging literature regarding individual CBT interventions for children with anxiety and ASD (e.g., Wood et al., 2015), and we would recommend that you research this area further before embarking on using this program with parents of children with ASD and anxiety difficulties.

Are the Child and/or Parent Motivated to Overcome the Anxiety Problem?

As emphasized in Chapter 1, the motivation and engagement of the parent is paramount to successfully delivering this treatment. If the child is not particularly motivated to overcome his or her anxiety, this is something you can address with the parent as part of this intervention and is thus not a reason to forgo embarking on a parent-based CBT intervention. In fact, it is an advantage of this particular approach. If the parent does not appear motivated to work on the child's anxiety, this low parental motivation poses a bigger problem. Some parents request that their child be seen individually because they feel that they will be unable to resolve the child's issues themselves. Indeed, we have found that when families are offered a choice between parent-led CBT and individual CBT with the child, they often express a preference for child to be seen, hoping that the therapist will "fix" him or her. However, when a parent-led approach is offered as the routine first line of treatment, the uptake is high, good outcomes are achieved, and parents are highly satisfied. Indeed, some parents have reflected to us that they were initially cautious about the approach, but having been through the process, they feel that their whole family has benefited. This feedback highlights the need to clearly explain the rationale for this approach and its potential advantages. As such, we would suggest that you take the following steps:

- Emphasize that the program is about the child and not them (as there is often a misunderstanding about the focus of treatment).
- Enable the parent to fully understand the treatment model (see Chapter 3).

- Highlight the efficiency of the intervention (reduced number of sessions as compared to child-directed CBT).
- Emphasize the effectiveness of parent-led interventions (e.g., Thirlwall et al., 2013).
- Provide anecdotal evidence from other parents who have held similar concerns prior to treatment.
- Encourage the parent to give the approach a try, with agreement to review progress carefully throughout treatment.

Are the Parents in a Position to Attend Regular Sessions and to Access the Strategies Outlined in This Book in a Way That Will Enable Them to Make Progress?

It is important to emphasize the need for regular contact between the therapist and the parent, although these contacts do not have to all be face to face but can also be conducted on the phone. It is also important to assess whether you feel that the parent will be able to understand and implement the strategies contained in this book. We do not typically assess these issues formally, but the level of parental literacy is an important consideration. Questions about parental literacy need to be asked sensitively, as mentioned previously; for example, "Are you comfortable with reading treatment materials between sessions?" If parental literacy presents an issue for the family, the following strategies may be useful:

- Ask the parent to identify a friend/family member who can support him or her in reading the material and implementing the strategies.
- Ask the parent to identify a friend/family member to attend the sessions in order to provide support.
- Take more time to explain strategies and to clarify understanding (may require increased number of sessions).
- Audio-record sessions and give the recording to the parent at the end of each session.
- Provide a written summary of each session to the parent, with key points highlighted.
- Use flashcards to record key points for parents and/or for homework tasks.

Setting Goals for Treatment

Once it has been established that anxiety is the child's primary problem, we recommend that therapists consider what it is that the child and/or parent

wants to work toward changing and help him or her to identify treatment
goals.

Setting goals is an important component of treatment because it
directs attention and effort toward relevant activities, provides structure to
the treatment, promotes collaboration, provides an objective target against
which to measure progress, and engenders a sense of hope and control
(Locke & Latham, 2002). Early agreement between the therapist and the
client on goals has been associated with subsequent clinical improvement
(e.g., Safran & Wallner, 1991). Therapist–client agreement on goals is also
a key component of the working alliance in therapy, which has been found
to be related positively to outcomes across different types of therapy (e.g.,
Horvath, Del Re, Flückiger, & Symonds, 2011).

Although goal setting may seem fairly straightforward, it can sometimes be difficult for parents to identify clear goals. Understandably parents often come to treatment with what they *don't* want their child to be
feeling or doing (e.g., "I don't want him or her to be scared any more") at
the front of their minds, but these ideas are difficult to measure and do
not equate to specific goals toward which the family can work. A useful
way of helping parents to turn these more general ambitions into goals is
to help them to unpack what achieving these might look like. It is also
important to distinguish between short-, medium-, and long-term goals.
The aim would ordinarily be to achieve short- and medium-term goals
within the time scale of the treatment sessions, and the parent and child
could continue to work toward longer-term goals following the end of the
sessions.

Useful Questions to Ask Parents

➤ "If [the child] was no longer anxious, what would he or she be
  doing differently? What difference would that make?"

➤ "What would [the child] be doing that he or she is currently
  unable to do because of anxiety?"

➤ "What changes would you/your partner notice?"

SMART is a useful acronym to aid in setting goals that are *specific, measurable, attainable, realistic,* and within a defined *time frame* (see Table 2.1).

Table 2.2 illustrates how general goals have been turned into more specific goals using SMART principles.

TABLE 2.1. Goal-Setting Considerations

Is it specific?

Parents may need help to identify specific achievements that will show that progress has been made.

Is it measurable?

It should be clear as to when the goal has been achieved.

Is it achievable?

The goal needs to be something that the child can actually achieve. For example, some goals may require others to be available (e.g., staying over at grandparents) or an outing to be planned (e.g., going on an airplane that requires the family to book a holiday).

Is it realistic?

The goal needs to be in line with reality. For example, expecting a child who is currently socially anxious to become the most outgoing child in his or her school would not be realistic.

What time frame should be given?

Parents should aim to have a clear amount of time in mind as to when the goal needs to be achieved. This should be realistic so that parents don't become frustrated or give up if the goal cannot be achieved in that time.

TABLE 2.2. Turning General Goals into Specific Goals

Vague goal	SMART goal
"For x to be less anxious."	"For x to stay over at her grandparents without us by the end of this treatment."
"For x to make friends."	"For x to ask someone from his class over to our house in the next 3 weeks."
"For x to enjoy school again."	"For x to go to all of her classes within the next 2 months."
"For x to worry less."	"For x to be in bed asleep by 10:00 P.M. on school nights by the end of this month."
"For x to stop avoiding dogs."	"For x to walk past a dog in the street without crossing the road within the next 3 weeks."

Reviewing Progress

Goals need to be reviewed on a regular basis to keep focused and to identify progress that has been made. Reviewing goals regularly helps parents
stay on track and sometimes also engenders hope by helping parents notice
changes. A simple method of reviewing goals includes asking parents to
identify on a scale of 0–10 how far they have moved toward achieving the
goal (0 = no progress at all, 10 = achieved the goal completely). This scale
system is also a useful way of tracking change throughout the treatment
process. Through these discussions, parents are sometimes surprised that
some progress has been made even in areas where they felt things had not
changed at all.

TAKE-HOME MESSAGES

✓ A comprehensive assessment of child anxiety difficulties requires
   information to be obtained in a range of different ways (interviews,
   questionnaires, observations) from multiple informants.

✓ Assessment should be focused and clearly targeted to gather
   comprehensive data about anxiety and any contributory factors.

✓ The burden of assessment imposed on the family must be manageable.

✓ A well-planned assessment will be invaluable and will serve to increase
   the chances of an effective intervention and positive outcomes.

✓ Treatment goals should be set collaboratively with parents and
   monitored throughout treatment.

CHAPTER 3

Psychoeducation and Individualizing the Treatment Model

The treatment approach we describe in this book follows a cognitive-behavioral approach. In other words, treatment focuses on the thoughts and behaviors that are maintaining the child's difficulties. This chapter provides an overview of the theoretical rationale for each part of the treatment covered in this book. As such, this chapter may feel a little heavier than the other chapters of the book; however, we urge you to stick with it because it is really important that both therapists and parents start treatment with a clear understanding of the purpose of each aspect of the treatment so that they can work together to consider how each aspect applies to individual children.

Understandably, parents typically come to treatment with many questions about why their child has developed problems with anxiety, often accompanied by guilt or negative feelings about things they feel that they or others have done that may have contributed to the problem. Equally, parents may be concerned that the therapist will make assumptions that they, as parents, are somehow to blame for their child's difficulties. We find it helpful to provide parents with an opportunity to express their concerns about the potential causes of their child's difficulties, and to enhance their understanding on the basis of what is known from empirical research.

This chapter starts with a brief overview of what is known about the development of anxiety disorders in children. We then review what we know about maintenance factors, before concluding with practical guidance on how to communicate some basic ideas to parents and how to work with parents to develop a shared understanding of the development and maintenance of their child's difficulties.

The Development of Anxiety Disorders in Children

Elsewhere we have suggested that key mechanisms in the development of child anxiety include (1) an anxious predisposition, (2) restricted opportunities or particular negative experiences, and/or (3) learning from others (Murray, Creswell, & Cooper, 2009; Creswell et al., 2015). This section briefly considers each of these factors.

Anxious Predisposition

Twin and adoption studies have shown that genetic factors are likely to have some influence on the development of childhood anxiety (Gregory & Eley, 2007), although there is not, as yet, a clear understanding of specific genetic factors that underlie anxiety. However, it is likely that these factors will differ in their effects depending on the environment that the child experiences (e.g., Fox et al., 2005). The trait that has been most extensively explored as indicating possible vulnerability for the development of anxiety is behavioral inhibition (BI), which is characterized by fear or withdrawal in response to novel or unfamiliar situations (e.g., meeting new people). Young children who exhibit high BI are more likely to develop anxiety disorders later in childhood, particularly social anxiety disorder (e.g., Hirshfeld-Becker, Micco, Simoes, & Henin, 2008). However, it is important to note that the risk associated with BI may only be realized when children experience particular environments. For example, Rubin, Burgess, and Hastings (2002) found that young children who were highly inhibited were only classified as shy as they got older if their mothers had been controlling or negative toward them (see "Parental Responses" on page 47 for more on parental responses).

Opportunities and Experiences

There has not been a great deal of research on the effects of early socialization experiences among children with anxiety disorders. However, some suggestive evidence has come from the Reading Longitudinal Study, in which we found that infants who experienced less caregiving by people other than the mothers (including the father) at 10 and 14 months of age experienced greater sleep problems at 2 years of age—a potential marker of later emotional problems (Creswell, Cooper, & Murray, 2010). These preliminary findings suggest that the opportunities that caregivers create for children to experience novelty and challenge may influence later child adjustment.

It has been suggested that the experience of negative life events may also put children at risk for developing anxiety disorders. Again, research is limited. However, Allen, Rapee, and Sandberg (2008) reported that mothers of children with anxiety disorders reported more discrete negative life events and chronic adversities in the 12 months prior to the onset of their child's disorder than mothers of nonanxious controls. Furthermore, the inclusion of objective raters of the impact of particular life events highlighted that the findings did not appear to be accounted for by potential biases in maternal reports.

Learning from Others

Learning theories have emphasized two pathways to the development of anxiety: (1) learning through observing others and (2) learning through receiving information from others. Experimental studies have provided evidence that children develop fears through observing the reactions of others. For example, children who observe their parent displaying fearful responses to potentially physical (e.g., toy snakes; Gerull & Rapee, 2002) or social (e.g., strangers; de Rosnay, Cooper, Tsigaras, & Murray, 2006) threats become more fearful when they themselves are confronted with these objects or situations. These findings have been supported by longitudinal studies in which higher maternal expressed anxiety, when the infant was 10–12 months of age, was associated with greater infant avoidance at a later assessment, particularly for children who had been identified as highly inhibited behaviorally (Murray et al., 2008; Aktar, Majdandžić, de Vente & Bögels, 2013). These findings highlight the particular impact that caregiver responses might have when the child has a more anxious temperament.

A number of experimental studies have shown that children's fearful beliefs and responses increase after they are given negative information by researchers (e.g., Field & Lawson, 2003) or by parents (e.g., Muris, van Zwol, Huijding, & Mayer, 2010; Remmerswaal, Muris, Mayer, & Smeets, 2010). In these studies children have typically been given positive, negative, or neutral information about unfamiliar animals and are then asked to rate their fearful beliefs and approach the animals. The findings align with studies from developmental psychology that have highlighted that children pick up opinions and beliefs from their parents, through both tuition and spontaneous conversations (e.g., Fivush, 1991; Nelson, 1993).

The Impact of Parental Anxiety on the Development of Child Anxiety

Because anxiety is known to commonly run in families, both parents and therapists can be concerned about the applicability of following a parent-led approach to treatment in the context of high parental anxiety. Therefore, we now briefly consider the potential impact of high parental anxiety on each of the factors that have been implicated in the development of child anxiety (also see Chapter 11).

Children of parents with anxiety disorders are at increased risk of developing psychiatric disorders (e.g., Beidel & Turner, 1997; Merikangas, Avenevoli, Dierker, & Grillon, 1999), particularly anxiety disorders, where the risk to children is four times higher than for offspring of parents who don't have an anxiety disorder (Micco et al., 2009). The mechanisms underlying this remain unclear, but recent findings suggest that shared genetic factors may not be the primary explanation (Eley et al., 2015). Indeed, it is possible that high levels of parental anxiety may increase the likelihood that each of the environmental pathways already mentioned will lead to the development of child anxiety. For example, in the case of socialization, highly anxious parents may place limits on their child's attempts to engage in wider experiences. In line with this possibility, we found that infants of mothers with social anxiety disorder were less likely to have received care from people other than the mother (Creswell, Cooper, et al., 2010). In addition, parental anxiety may be associated with increased exposure to particular negative life events that may affect the child. For example, adults with anxiety disorders are known to experience more negative life events, such as marital breakdown, than nonanxious adults (e.g., Kessler, Davis, & Kendler, 1997; Merikangas et al., 1999). It seems plausible to assume that highly anxious parents will also be more likely to model anxiety or express anxiety-promoting information. These assumptions have been supported by recent evidence that mothers with social anxiety disorder express higher levels of anxiety in a social challenge (Murray et al., 2008; Aktar et al., 2013) and make more catastrophic (Moore, Whaley, & Sigman, 2004) and threat-related comments (e.g., "That is terrifying!") and less encouragement (Murray et al., 2014) than nonanxious mothers. With these findings in mind, we discuss the application of parent-led CBT for child anxiety disorders in the context of high parental anxiety further in Chapter 11.

The development of child anxiety is likely to be influenced by a range of factors that interact with each other, including (1) an anxious predisposition, (2) restricted opportunities or particular negative experiences, and (3) learning from others. Some of these risk factors may be more likely to occur when there is a family history of anxiety.

The Maintenance of Anxiety Disorders in Children

CBT differs from many other psychological therapies in its focus on what is *maintaining* the problem. When working with children, it is sometimes difficult to distinguish between factors that account for development and those that are continuing to maintain the problem. For example, learning from observing others' responses influences the learning of fear responses, but it is equally likely that parents of anxious children will show signs of concern when their child faces a challenge because of their experiences as a child struggling with similar situations in the past. In this way, parental behaviors may be a response to the child's anxiety but may also inadvertently maintain the problem. In a similar vein, the potential maintenance factors outlined below may well have a developmental role, for example, if anxious children have a preexisting way of thinking about the world that puts them at risk of developing problems with anxiety. Future research is needed to establish the role of the factors described below in the development of anxiety disorders in children. For now, we focus on their potential role in the maintenance of child anxiety disorders and the implications for treatment.

Negative Expectations

A central idea behind cognitive theories of anxiety in adults is that anxious individuals have a tendency to infer future threat or danger in their environment and to underestimate their ability to cope. It is suggested that this thinking style leads to physiological arousal and behavioral avoidance, which in turn acts to keep anxiety going by preventing new learning (Beck & Clark, 1997). As such, biases in attention and interpretation that may reflect a tendency to notice and evaluate experiences in a threatening way have received particular research attention.

In terms of attention biases, cognitive-behavioral models hypothesize that a tendency to preferentially attend to anxiety-relevant stimuli in the environment exacerbates symptoms when an individual is under stress (e.g., Beck & Clark, 1997; Teasdale, 1988). In support of this theory, highly anxious, compared to low anxious, adults are quicker to look toward angry faces (threat stimuli) than neutral faces (e.g., Bar-Haim, Lamy, Pergamin, Bakermans-Kranenburg, & van IJzendoorn, 2007). Attention biases have also been examined among children and adolescents. However, findings to date have been somewhat inconsistent; some studies have found that highly anxious young people are more drawn to threat (e.g., Roy-Byrne et al., 2008), and others have found that they appear to avoid threat (e.g., Monk et al., 2006). Given the differences in findings, the implications for treatment remain unclear, and studies that have set out to alter attention biases in children with anxiety disorders have been inconclusive (e.g., Pennant et al., 2015). Recent findings have suggested that whether children attend to or away from threat stimuli may vary between specific anxiety and mood disorders, with attention away from threat being more relevant in phobic disorders and attention toward threat being more relevant in disorders characterized by rumination, such as GAD (Salum et al., 2013). For now, the implications for treatment remain unclear.

A tendency to interpret ambiguous information in an overly threatening way (Amir, Beard, & Bower, 2005; Mathews & Mackintosh, 2000) has also been implicated in the maintenance of anxiety disorders in adults. A number of studies have demonstrated that children and adolescents with anxiety disorders interpret ambiguous situations in a more negative manner than nonanxious young people (e.g., Barrett, Dadds & Rapee, 1996; Creswell, Schniering, & Rapee, 2005). For example, when presented with hypothetical situations where it is not clear what is happening (e.g., "Your teacher has been asking other children where you are"), children and adolescents with anxiety disorders are more likely to see the situation as negative ("She thinks I have done something wrong"). Change in anxious self-statements (e.g., "I am very nervous") has also been found to relate to treatment outcomes (Kendall & Treadwell, 2007). However, these studies have typically grouped together young people across fairly broad age ranges (e.g., 7–14 years; Barrett et al., 1996) and/or used measures that may not distinguish clearly from measures of anxiety symptoms (e.g., Kendall & Treadwell, 2007). Thus, the nature of thinking styles in children with anxiety disorders and the role of those styles in maintaining anxiety problems remains unclear.

We certainly might anticipate that the association between thinking styles and anxiety will differ across childhood and adolescence, as young people have more experiences to draw on and as thinking styles become more stable and global (e.g., Nolen-Hoeksema, Girgus, & Seligman, 1992). In keeping with this likelihood, studies limited to 7- to 12-year-olds have varied in what they have found about the association between threat interpretation and anxiety disorders, with some studies finding significant differences between children with and without anxiety disorders (e.g., Alkozei et al., 2014; Waters, Wharton, Zimmer-Gembeck, & Craske, 2008) and others not (Creswell, Murray, & Cooper, 2014; Waters, Craske, Bergman, & Treanor, 2008; Waite, Codd, & Creswell, 2015). Instead it has been suggested that, in childhood, an underestimation of one's ability to cope with potentially difficult situations may play a more central role in the maintenance of anxiety than thoughts focused on threat or danger (e.g., Alfano, Beidel, & Turner, 2002; Creswell & O'Connor, 2011; Waters, Wharton, et al., 2008), although this association may also vary across this developmental stage (Creswell et al., 2014; Waite et al., 2015). Recent findings from a large U.S. multicenter trial of treatments for anxiety disorders in children and adolescents indicate that improvements in children's coping abilities (but not negative thinking styles) accounted for positive treatment outcomes (Kendall et al., 2016), suggesting that enhancing coping abilities and/or perceptions may be a critical part of treatment.

All in all, there remains a lack of clarity about whether, how, and what kind of thinking styles are involved in the maintenance of anxiety problems in preadolescent children. Indeed, we have recently found that in middle childhood there may be a general tendency to interpret ambiguous situations as threatening, whether children are anxious or not (Waite et al., 2015). What seems to be critical is how anxious children then respond to this potential threat, for example, by developing ways of coping or by engaging in avoidance (see "Anxious or Avoidant Behaviors" on page 46). For this reason we have moved away from an explicit focus on helping children to logically evaluate threat-based thoughts in order to generate "positive" or "helpful" thoughts within treatment. Instead, we focus on helping children develop curiosity about possible outcomes in order to encourage them to approach situations they would otherwise avoid as a way to learn new things about themselves or the situation. This approach is in line with recent experimental studies with adults (e.g., Craske et al., 2014) that have suggested that facing feared stimuli is more effective when people's negative expectations are violated by the exposure. In other words, the exposure provides an opportunity to learn something new. In contrast, when people engage in activities to generate more positive expectations prior to the exposure, then the opportunity for experiential learning is reduced (and the exposure ultimately less successful) because they are not learning anything new or surprising. This change in approach has also been encouraged by our work with both therapists and families. We have often found that that by explicitly setting out to help children develop "positive" or "helpful" thoughts, children can end up feeling like they are being coerced or not being listened to, which can be frustrating for both the child and their parent/therapist; and if new thoughts are generated, they are less likely to be sufficiently strong to "stick." For all these reasons we do not include strategies in this book to help children develop "positive" thoughts prior to exposure. However, we do recognize that if a child's tendency is to respond to his or her negative expectations with avoidance, then it may be strategically useful (i.e., encourage a willingness in the child to engage in exposure) to help the child develop a sense of curiosity about these expectations and be open to the possibility that other outcomes might occur. We describe this mental state as "have a go" thinking, and we describe it further in Chapter 5.

Anxious or Avoidant Behaviors

Avoidance of feared situations or objects is a central feature of anxiety disorders. Although avoidance is an understandable reaction to fear, cognitive-behavioral theories suggest that it can also maintain the problem by preventing new learning about the actual danger posed by the situation and/or about one's ability to tolerate the associated discomfort. Children with anxiety disorders typically present with a range of avoidant behaviors: for example, sleeping with their parent rather than alone, not answering questions in class, or staying away from particular animals. In all these cases, children do not have the opportunity to learn, for example, that they will be OK in their own bed, that they can cope when they get the wrong answer, or that there are things that they can do that can make dogs less likely to jump up (and that they can cope if they do). However, children (more than adults) may at times be forced into particular feared situations that they don't have the choice to actively avoid; for example, separating from their parent to go to class. In these situations children may become highly distressed, which may strengthen the original belief by enhancing learning that, for example, separating from a parent feels horrible. As such, treatment focuses on helping children to overcome avoidance in a managed and supported way in which they can tolerate the associated discomfort. A number of studies have highlighted that managed exposure to feared stimuli is particularly critical to successful treatment outcomes. For example, Peris et al. (2015) reported that the onset of exposure within CBT for child anxiety disorders leads to a greater reduction in anxiety severity than other treatment components (relaxation and cognitive restructuring), particularly in preadolescent children. We discuss how to help parents successfully engage their children in exposure and how to optimize the new learning that takes place in Chapter 6.

Parental Responses

The parental behaviors that have most commonly been linked to child-hood anxiety disorders are parental control and negativity. Parental control, intrusiveness, overprotection, and lack of autonomy promotion have not, on the whole, been clearly distinguished in the literature. However, the general suggestion is that if parents excessively regulate children's behavior and discourage independence, then they are likely to (1) communicate to their children that the world is a dangerous and uncontrollable place (e.g., Hudson & Rapee, 2004), and (2) prevent the children from developing a sense of competence and mastery, instead reinforcing their tendency to avoid challenges (Chorpita & Barlow, 1998). Furthermore, it is suggested that parents who respond to their children with negativity may lead them to believe that the environment is fundamentally hostile and threatening and that outcomes will be negative, promoting a sense of low self-worth and competence (Parker, 1983). Cross-sectional studies in which the association between these sorts of parenting behaviors and anxiety are examined at any one point in time have provided support for a significant association between overcontrol and child anxiety, although evidence for an association with parental negativity has been less compelling (e.g., Mcleod, Weisz, & Wood, 2007).

A difficulty with cross-sectional studies is that they cannot tell us which factor (if any) influences the other. When it comes to parental overcontrol, observations of parents interacting with anxious and nonanxious children highlight how parents change their behaviors *in response to* the child's anxiety. Specifically, parents tended to be more controlling in their interactions with anxious than nonanxious children, regardless of whether they were their own children (Hudson, Doyle, & Gar, 2009). On the other hand, there is also evidence that parents who are trained to be more controlling provoke heightened anxiety in their children when they face a challenge (de Wilde & Rapee, 2008), particularly if these children have high levels of trait anxiety (Thirlwall & Creswell, 2010). As such, parental overcontrol appears to have a potential role in a vicious cycle in which it is both a response and a reinforcer of child anxiety. For this reason, parents are encouraged and supported in promoting their child's independence throughout this program (in particular, see Chapter 4).

High levels of parental anxiety may also influence parental responses to children's anxiety. Specifically, we have found that mothers of anxious children, who had an anxiety disorder themselves, reported more negative expectations of their children, showed higher levels of intrusive and anxious behaviors and lower levels of warmth, and were more negative when interacting with their children than mothers without anxiety disorders, particularly when their children appeared visibly anxious during the task (Creswell, Apetroaia, Murray, & Cooper, 2013). These findings suggest that overcontrolling and (possibly) negative responses may reflect a common and potentially reinforcing response pattern to parenting an anxious or inhibited child, and that these behaviors may be especially likely to arise in parents who are themselves prone to anxiety and when their child is confronted by a challenge (see Chapter 11).

Our view is that particular responses are drawn out of parents by anxious children and are often a natural response to trying to help an anxious child. In addition, we recognize that these behaviors may be perfectly effective with other children who have different dispositions. Our aims, therefore, are to help parents develop a set of strategies, based on CBT, that will provide alternatives to these "natural responses" and help them in the challenging situations they have to manage due to having a highly anxious child. The majority of parents that we work with tell us that they feel guilty or to blame for their child's difficulties, and in many cases, professionals have reinforced this view. By taking a parent-led approach, there is a danger that parents will conclude that we must therefore think that "it's their fault." As we have noted in Chapter 1 and in this chapter, this impression is far from the truth, but it is clearly essential that discussions about parental factors must be sensitive to these parental concerns.

> Anxiety in children is likely to be maintained by a number of interacting factors, including how children and others around them respond to potential threat in the environment.

The Guiding Model

In summary, there are a number of potential pathways to childhood anxiety disorders, many of which present a risk only if they co-occur with another risk factor (e.g., particular experiences in the context of a particular temperament). Whereas there may be a general tendency among preadolescent children to interpret ambiguity in a relatively negative way, children who are highly anxious appear to respond to negative expectations with a sense that they won't be able to cope and therefore with avoidance or distress. These responses often provoke parental responses that may inadvertently promote avoidance rather than encouraging children to approach the situations they fear. Figure 3.1 illustrates this process in diagrammatic form. This model will no doubt change as further understanding develops, but

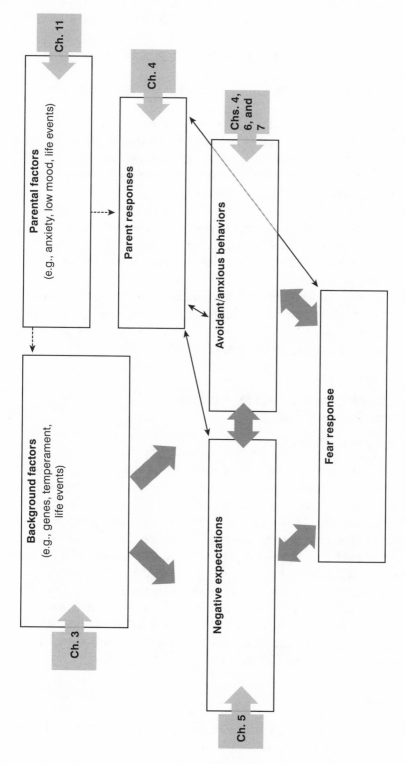

FIGURE 3.1. A general model to guide treatment.

we have found it a useful guide in informing how we work with parents of anxious children.

Specifically, the strategies that we describe in this book aim to:

- Provide psychoeducation both about the treatment model and potential developmental factors in order for parents to update their understanding of their child's difficulties with anxiety (this chapter).
- Encourage parental responses that promote independence and a willingness to "have a go" (Chapter 4).
- Guide parents in helping their child to develop curiosity about his or her thoughts and to encourage willingness to test them out (Chapter 5).
- Guide parents in helping their children to engage in exposure to create opportunities for new learning through facing and testing their fears (Chapter 6).
- Help parents develop problem-solving skills that they can use themselves to (1) effectively put this program in place, and (2) apply with their child to encourage independent problem solving (as an alternative to relying on parents to step in) (Chapter 7).

Communicating the Rationale for Treatment to Parents: Psychoeducation

What the Evidence Tells Us

Psychoeducation is a key aspect of many psychological therapies, particularly CBT, and there is some evidence that it can improve psychological functioning in its own right (e.g., Donker, Griffiths, Cuijpers, & Christensen, 2009). In the context of this treatment, the primary aims of psychoeducation are (1) to aid the parent's (and ultimately the child's) understanding of the symptoms that the child experiences and how these can be targeted in treatment; (2) to clarify misconceptions about the problem or the treatment (e.g., that the parent is to blame); (3) to alleviate stress and negative affect (potentially caused by misconceptions, e.g., guilt); (4) to enhance the parent's (and child's) sense of control over the child's difficulties; and (5) to promote the parent's and child's use of the strategies introduced in the treatment (e.g., see Chan, Richardson & Richardson, 2011).

What Are the Goals?

Table 3.1 outlines the key aims of psychoeducation and the themes that are important to cover in relation to each goal.

TABLE 3.1. Goals and Themes of Psychoeducation

Goals	Themes
To promote parental understanding of possible maintaining factors and the treatment model, and to consider together how they apply to this individual child.	• Description of the anxiety cycle • Listening carefully to the parents throughout • Individualizing the treatment model
To provide the rationale for each element of the program and to promote use of the treatment strategies	• Highlighting the strategies that relate to each part of the anxiety cycle
To provide an opportunity for parents to express their views about the causes of their child's difficulties and to provide parents with an opportunity to enhance their knowledge about the causes of anxiety	• Appreciation of parental perspectives, insight, and knowledge • Provision of overview of what is known about the development of anxiety • Emphasis on the interactive nature of risk factors • Emphasis on the responses from others that child anxiety may provoke

How to Do It

Psychoeducation is inevitably fairly didactic in parts, with the therapist conveying information to support each of the preceding goals. However, it is equally important to use this phase of treatment to work together with the parent to think about the rationale for treatment and the treatment model in relation to the individual child. It is therefore essential to reflect on whether and how the information presented relates to this particular child and his or her difficulties. Here we provide some guidance on how to get the information across in a way that maximizes parental engagement and involvement. We find that using a shared diagram representing the treatment model can provide a useful structure for discussions about the treatment model, its rationale, and its implications.

Handout 3.1* provides a diagram that can be filled in with information describing the individual child's experience. Figure 3.2 is a completed example for James, a 9-year-old boy with a specific fear of dogs.

---

*All reproducible handouts are at the ends of chapters.

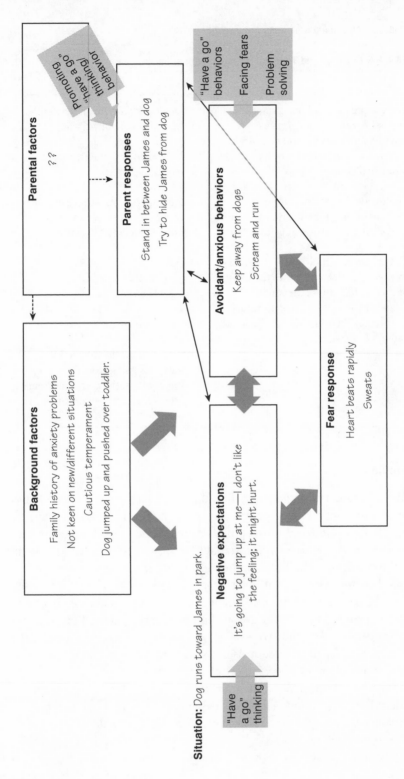

FIGURE 3.2. James's model and treatment guide.

Providing Information about the Nature of Anxiety

A good starting point is to complete the maintenance cycle of anxiety (in Handout 3.1) with the parent focusing on the child's negative expectations, fear responses, and avoidant/anxious behaviors. Here we describe these core sets of symptoms and their potential role in maintaining anxiety—specifically, that children of this age often have a tendency to see the world in a threatening way, which can lead to avoidance or distress in highly anxious children. By referring to a specific situation that would elicit anxiety in the child, we ask the parent to hypothesize about the child's thoughts, behaviors, and fear response and to use this information to provide a rationale for each of the elements of treatment. A sample conversation follows.

THERAPIST: Many children of James's age are likely to expect that something bad is going to happen when they go into situations that are new or when they are not sure what is going to happen. [*Providing rationale for the question.*] You told me that the park is a particularly hard place for James to go to. What sorts of things does James think will happen if it goes to the park? [*Asking questions to individualize the model. Focusing on a specific situation.*]

PARENT: Well, it's all about dogs, really. You never know if you'll see a dog or not, but he doesn't want to take the risk.

THERAPIST: What does he think will happen if he sees a dog? [*Gathering information about specific thoughts.*]

PARENT: I'm not really sure, but I think it's really about them jumping up, because that happened to him when he was quite small. It was a big dog, so it pushed him over and it really gave him a fright. Since then, he won't go near them.

THERAPIST: OK. So you can check this out with James before we meet next time, [*Setting up need to gather information from the child between sessions.*] but for now, let's assume that it's the possibility that a dog might jump up that he's worried about. I can appreciate that that might not be nice, [*Acknowledging the child's fear response.*] but what exactly about a dog jumping up do you think he doesn't like? [*Gathering more details about specific thoughts.*]

PARENT: Well, he hasn't been bitten before, and I don't really think that that is what he is thinking about. It's more that it really gave him a shock, and he really didn't like that. I suppose he might be worried that it would hurt if he got pushed right over or maybe if the dog scratched him.

THERAPIST: OK. Great. That's all really helpful information. [*Reinforcing the parent's response.*] Let's jot that down [see Figure 3.2]. [*Record keeping.*] What we also know from research that has been done is that children who have particular problems with anxiety are less likely to think that they can cope with challenging situations like this, and it sounds like that might be the case for James. Do you think that's right? [*Checking out whether this aspect of theory applies to James.*]

PARENT: Yes, definitely. I'm not sure how likely he thinks these things are to happen, but he just thinks he couldn't deal with it if something like that did happen.

THERAPIST: OK. So what he does in that sort of situation seems to make lots of sense, doesn't it? [*Making links between child's thoughts and behaviors.*]

PARENT: Yes, basically he just tries to stay away from anywhere that he might come across a dog—or if we do accidentally end up in a situation where there is a dog, he completely freaks out and starts screaming and tries to run away.

THERAPIST: OK. Let's jot that down too. And do you notice any other signs that he is feeling anxious? [*Eliciting description of fear response.*]

PARENT: He just gets really panicky; he says that his heart beats fast and his hands go all sweaty. It's really horrible for him [recorded on Figure 3.2].

THERAPIST: Yes, it does really sound horrible. And what do you think he learns from that? [*Eliciting potential maintenance cycle.*]

PARENT: It's just another reason to stay away from dogs, isn't it? It's just such a horrible experience every time we see one.

THERAPIST: So that really feeds in to his sense that seeing dogs will be horrible for him [highlighting feedback arrow on Figure 3.2]. [*Specifying maintenance cycle.*] It sounds like it must be pretty hard going for you or whoever is with him too? [*Eliciting parent's response.*]

PARENT: Yes, definitely. If we are out and I spot a dog, I'll try to block it from his view or distract him so he doesn't see it. Or if one actually comes near us, I'll stand between James and the dog so it can't go near him, because I don't want him to start running and put himself in danger.

THERAPIST: Yes, of course. So let's jot that down here [Figure 3.2]. So we can see how your responses are a pretty natural response to James's reaction. [*Normalizing parental response.*] What do you think James learns from those responses? [*Eliciting potential maintenance cycle.*]

PARENT: Well, hopefully that I'll protect him if need be.

THERAPIST: And what does he learn about his own ability to cope? [*Eliciting potential maintenance cycle.*]

PARENT: (*Laughs.*) Ah, I see what you mean. Well, that he can't—but I can't really let him go running out of the park screaming, can I? There are really busy roads all around, and he gets in such a state. Once he almost got run over because he's just not thinking straight.

THERAPIST: That sounds terrifying, [*Acknowledging the parent's feelings.*] and, of course, it's going to be a completely natural reaction [*Normalizing the parent's response.*] to try to protect him, but the problem is that our natural reactions don't always give opportunities for our children to learn new things—for example, how to cope in the situation. You are also right that we can't let him run screaming out of the park, as that isn't going to be a good learning experience for him either and could even be dangerous. So we will be working together to figure out some ways that will help James face his fears and learn new things about dogs and about himself—but gradually and with support. How does that sound? [*Provide rationale for approach and check it out with the parent.*]

PARENT: We can try.

THERAPIST: We will be working together to deal which most of the parts of this picture [Figure 3.2]. First of all, we want to start to help James think about things in a way that prepares him to have a go at facing his fears [indicate on Figure 3.2]. Then we'll be working on ways that help him feel more confident about having a go at things that are new or that he's not comfortable with, including facing his fears [indicate on Figure 3.2]. Things aren't always going to go right, and sometimes we might face obstacles to making this all work, so we'll also spend some time helping you both to solve problems along the way [indicate on Figure 3.2]. Working together on these areas and using all of these strategies will help you feel equipped to support James in overcoming these difficulties [indicate on Figure 3.2]. How does that sound to you? [*Provide rationale for approach and check it out with the parent.*]

As illustrated in the preceding dialogue, it can be important to start to consider the potential maintaining role of other people's responses to the child in order to guide you in the focus of treatment. For example, one parent may tend to reassure his or her child in response to heightened anxiety, another may struggle to encourage the child's independence, and still another may tend to step in when the child begins to struggle for fear that the child will not be able to cope or just out of frustration and to "get on with it." As we have already highlighted, parents are likely to be concerned that you are blaming them for their child's difficulties, so it is critical that a clear rationale is provided to parents for this line of questioning. In our experience "beating around the bush" or introducing these sorts of questions in an apologetic way can make parents feel that the therapist is being disingenuous. These sorts of questions can be introduced helpfully to parents in the following way:

"It is really helpful for me to get a sense of how you respond when your child gets anxious. You are no doubt doing some really helpful things, and that is really important for me to be aware of so that I can encourage you to put those strategies into place at other times when they might be helpful. We also know that having an anxious child can make parenting really difficult, because children can draw responses out of us that might inadvertently get in the way of helping them overcome their difficulties. Knowing about these responses can help us to work together to develop alternatives that might help them move forward in overcoming anxiety."

Useful Questions to Ask Parents

➤ "How do you typically respond to your child when he or she is anxious? Can you give an example of a recent incident?"

➤ "When your child gets anxious, what sorts of things does the child want you to do for him or her?"

➤ "What do you do when your child wants to avoid something that he or she finds anxiety-provoking—for example, going to school or to a party? Can you tell me about a time when that has happened recently?"

➤ "How do other members of your family respond at these times? Again, can you give me a recent example?"

It is critical that when they describe how they react to their child, parents receive an understanding response that acknowledges how difficult it can be to parent a child when he or she is highly anxious. If a parent describes reassuring the child (e.g., "Don't worry, it will all be fine"), for example, we might say the following:

"Lots of parents with whom I have worked tell me that they would generally reassure their child that everything is OK and that nothing bad will happen, just as you have described. This is a completely natural response that we all do from time to time, and it can work well for many children. Highly anxious children are likely to be seeking reassurance from us a great deal of the time. Do you find that this is a helpful response for your child? Do you find that reassuring him or her is usually enough, or do you find yourself having to provide reassurance about the same thing again and again?"

"[If yes] Yes, many parents tell us the same thing—that reassurance only seems to help in the short term. We'll be talking about some alternatives to reassurance in future sessions, so this is really useful for us to keep in mind."

 Sticking Point

The parents don't think the model fits for their child.

It is perfectly possible that some aspects of the model may not fit for any particular child, but we have very rarely encountered a situation where the parent cannot relate to some aspect of the model. We have also often found that when we present the model to parents, they may not immediately see the relevance to their child, but they may come back the following week, having collected information and having had an opportunity to reflect on the discussions, with clear examples of how the model fits for their child. In order to facilitate reflection, it is essential that the therapist present the model as a set of guiding principles that may or may not apply in any individual circumstance and foster a shared sense of curiosity in the parent and therapist.

If, even after reflection and information gathering, no aspect of the model seems to apply, then it will be important to review the assessment to confirm that anxiety is the child's primary presenting problem.

Providing Parents with an Opportunity to Express Their Views
about the Causes of Anxiety and to Update Their Knowledge

It is important to emphasize to parents that the treatment is going to focus on what is keeping the problem going now, and this is often not the same thing that led to the problem in the first place. For example, a child may have become fearful of going to school following a particular incident with some other children, but after being absent from school for some time, the problem may be kept going by the child's concerns that he or she won't now be able to cope with being behind on the work, having not maintained friendships, or how he or she will deal with questions about not having attended school in a while. Nonetheless, many parents are keen to talk about potential causes of their child's difficulties, and this can be important and useful to help them to see the potential for change.

> When talking to parents about what is known regarding the causes of anxiety in children, it is important to emphasize that anxiety difficulties are often a response to a combination of different factors that might include the child's temperament and particular experiences that he or she has had. We typically give a brief overview of the research evidence in lay terms and ask parents whether they feel this aspect of the research applies to their child.

It is certainly not the case that all of the areas identified in the research literature and described above apply to all the families we see. As shown in Figure 3.2, James's parents did not recognize any parental factors as having a causal role in the development of James's difficulties with dogs, so this part of the model was left blank. Sometimes we find that parents return to the following session having reflected on the model and volunteer additional information that they feel is relevant—but this will be information for them to convey, rather than for the therapist to assume is relevant or to impose upon them.

THERAPIST: We are not really going to be focusing on things that might have led to James's developing the problems in the first place [refer to Figure 3.2]. Instead we will be focusing on these parts of the drawing [refer to Figure 3.2] that are keeping James's fears going. But we do know that parents often have different thoughts and questions about what has caused their children's difficulties, and sometimes these can make it harder to focus solidly on the treatment, so it can be useful for us to talk about causes before we get started. [*Provide rationale for discussing causes and check it out with the parent.*] Does that sound OK?

PARENT: Well, yes. I mean, as you know, a massive dog did jump up at him when he was small, and that basically terrified him from then on.

THERAPIST: Yes, that certainly does sound frightening. [*Acknowledging the child's feellings.*] Do you think all children would have reacted in the same way? [*Inquire whether there may be other factors interacting with the child's experience to inform learning.*]

PARENT: Um, no, maybe not. I mean my younger child probably wouldn't bat an eyelid, to be honest. But James has always been the more cautious one, and he doesn't really like situations where he's not really sure what's going to happen. When he was younger, he didn't really like any big changes.

THERAPIST: That's interesting and certainly fits with what has been found in research about anxiety in children. There have been a number of studies that suggest that whether a child develops difficulties with anxiety or not is influenced by a combination of the child's temperament or personality, and his or her experiences. These experiences could be particular things, like the dog jumping up, and can also be how other people around the child respond in different situations. The difficulty is that not only are children who have a more anxious temperament more influenced by how other people respond around them, but they also behave in a way that makes us more likely to do certain things when we are with them. Does that seem to make sense to you? [*Reflect on relevant research literature and check it out with the parent.*]

PARENT: I'm not sure.

THERAPIST: A simple example would be to imagine a child who is terrified of clowns. The child might be on the lookout for messages from others about how safe he or she will be around clowns and might pick up on the slightest hint that clowns are a bad thing. But because we know the child is going to be terrified, when we see a clown we are likely to look concerned ourselves and might want to keep the child away from the clown to prevent any upset in the child. Can you see where this is going? [*Provide example to illustrate research literature and check it out with the parent.*]

PARENT: So, then the child picks up on that.

THERAPIST: Exactly. It's a really tricky situation to be in as parents because children pull certain responses out of us—but then they learn from those responses that they need to keep being scared. Whereas a much more laid-back child would be less likely to pull those responses out of us, and also might not pick up on how we behave in quite the same way. [*Acknowledging the difficulty of parenting an anxious child.*] Do you think this sort of idea fits for James? [*Check it out with the parent.*]

PARENT: Well, it's definitely true that I am quite different in how I do things with James compared to his brother, who is, like you say, much more laid back.

THERAPIST: Yes. Parenting an anxious child can be really challenging, particularly when you've no doubt been given lots of different advice from lots of different people. [*Acknowledging the difficulty of parenting an anxious child.*]

PARENT: That's right, everyone has an opinion.

THERAPIST: And it can also be even more challenging if we are quite anxious ourselves or have had particular experiences that affect how we parent. That's what this box refers to [Figure 3.2]. Do you think there is anything we should add in here? [*Introduce the parental factors component of the model and check it out with the parent.*]

PARENT: No. I can't really think of anything. None of the rest of us has ever had any problems like this. That's what makes it so weird.

THERAPIST: OK. We can leave this one blank [Figure 3.2]. [*Accept parental response.*] It sounds like you are saying that James is the only one in the family who experiences difficulties with anxiety? [*Check out parental views about transmission within the family.*]

PARENT: Well, no. None of us in our house do, but my husband's mother actually had enormous problems with anxiety. It does really worry me, as I don't want him to end up having the problems she has had—but I do also wonder if he has got it from her.

THERAPIST: That is something that parents often worry about understandably. Let's mark it down here under background factors [Figure 3.2]. Research on anxiety in children does tell us that there seems to be some genetic influence, but out of all the different things that do influence how anxious a child becomes, it seems that genes account for only about a third of them [*Provide information on genetic basis of anxiety in children and the potential gene–environment interaction.*] and that children's life experiences account for the rest.

As we talked about before, it also seems that even if a child has a predisposition to anxiety, whether it becomes a problem or not is heavily influenced by his or her experiences. So if we look at what we have noted in this picture [Figure 3.2], we can really understand why James reacts to dogs in the way he does. That understanding is going to really help us work together to come up with ways to help James have different sorts of experiences that will mean that, despite having a more cautious nature, anxiety will not get in the way of his life. How does that sound? [*Use model to provide rationale for the approach, keeping in mind potential predisposing factors.*]

 Sticking Points

The parent finds it hard to contribute to discussions about potential causal factors.

There are a number of reasons why parents may not feel comfortable reflecting on factors that may have influenced the development of their child's difficulties. As we have emphasized, parents may feel guilty or blamed, or there may be personal aspects of their history that they are not comfortable disclosing so early in their relationship with the therapist. This is all absolutely understandable, and as far as treatment is concerned, it is absolutely fine. Parents shouldn't be coerced in to these discussions. Rather, the empirical evidence should be presented as highlighting a number of potential routes to the development of anxiety in children, any of which may or may not apply to this individual child. Emphasize that the reason for covering this area is that many parents find it useful to have this context, but the treatment is primarily focused on what is keeping the problem going now (rather than what has happened before)—a focus with which the parent may be more comfortable. In short, the content and depth of these discussions can be guided by parents and what they might want to know. In practice, we find that some parents return to this conversation in a later session, when they have had time to think about the information.

The parents have different views on the cause or maintenance of their child's problems.

It is sometimes the case that two parents have different ideas about what is causing or maintaining their child's difficulties. In order to keep both parents engaged in treatment and help them to feel empowered in tackling their child's difficulties, it is important not to be drawn in to taking sides. Instead, it is critical to listen to and acknowledge both parents' points of views and to emphasize that anxiety difficulties often arise as an interaction of different factors (e.g., if one parent attributes the difficulties to genetics, and the other to parenting). It is important to be clear that ultimately, you will be treating these different views as hypotheses to be tested, which can only occur by fully engaging in the treatment approach.

The parents attribute the cause of their child's difficulties to something that is not supported by empirical evidence or that the therapist sees as irrelevant.

Again, this is fine. Of course we will never know with certainty what has led to this particular child's difficulties, but we can hypothesize about what is maintaining them and target these factors. The parent's perspective on this is essential. In order to move forwards, the parent will be helped the most by having an understanding of the child's difficulties that is compatible with the idea that change is possible. If the beliefs parents bring regarding the causes/maintenance of their child's difficulties are not consistent with this basic assumption about the possibility of change, it would be important to provide them with additional information from the research literature that they can add to their knowledge base to help them gradually move toward a position of hopefulness. For example, if a parent holds the view that the child was born this way and that is just how he or she is, it would be important to acknowledge that many children with anxiety disorders have an anxious or sensitive temperament, but that there is good evidence to suggest that children's experiences can make a difference as to whether this anxious temperament becomes a disorder and causes them problems in their day-to-day life. Through treatment, particular experiences can be created to maximize the chance of the child being able to make choices and enjoy his or her life.

TAKE-HOME MESSAGES

✓ The aim of psychoeducation is to provide information on the anxiety model in order to give a clear rationale for what you will cover in treatment.

✓ Providing the opportunity to consider what is known about causes of child anxiety difficulties can help reduce feelings of blame and promote a sense that change is possible.

✓ Collaboration is essential to ensure that both you and the parent fully understand the child's particular anxiety difficulties and to empower the parent to help the child tackle these difficulties.

HANDOUT 3.1. A Personalized Model to Guide Treatment

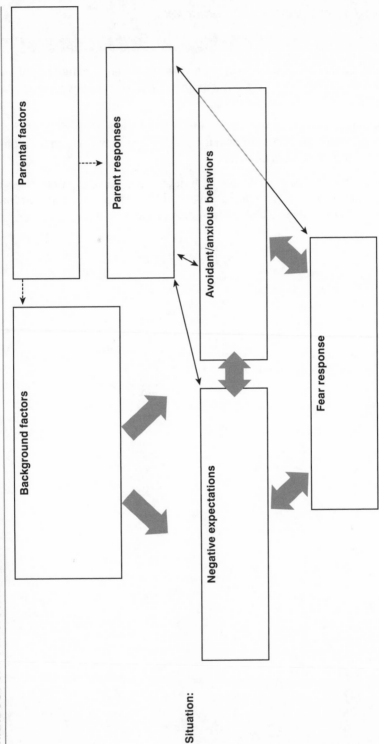

Situation:

CHAPTER 4

Promoting Independence in Day-to-Day Life

Anxious children often withdraw from trying new or challenging things. Although it may feel to them, and also possibly seem to others, that they are less able than other children, the fact is that they may well be no less durable or capable of acquiring new skills than their peers. Instead, what may set them apart from their peers is whether or not they are prepared to attempt challenges independently. As discussed in Chapter 3, for some anxious children, this aversion to challenges may partly be due to having an inhibited temperament that makes them more cautious in the face of new or unfamiliar things. However, a vicious cycle can arise in which holding back or relying on others can prevent the child from gaining opportunities to develop a sense of mastery and control, leading to ongoing anxiety. Few of us like to engage in an activity if we believe we won't be successful, but, for the most part, we learn through our experiences that setbacks and discomfort are transient, and with perseverance, many challenges can be overcome. A child who avoids trying difficult things misses out on valuable opportunities to develop this perspective.

From our observations and from talking to parents of anxious children, we know that stepping back and encouraging an anxious child to try things for him- or herself can feel counterintuitive. Anxious children often signal to others that they need assistance, and it is natural to want to help children when they show distress, particularly if an adult is anxious him- or herself. It can also seem quicker and easier to do things for these children. However, in order to increase children's sense of accomplishment and help them develop skills in dealing with problematic situations, it is important that they get the opportunity to practice being independent in a supported way. Part of being independent is feeling able to "have a go" and to give things a try even in the face of uncertainty. Parents can help their child to develop "have a go" responses to challenges by first building up their independence in nonemotive daily tasks before encouraging them to apply the same responses to situations that they find anxiety-provoking.

What the Evidence Tells Us

How Do Anxious Children View Themselves?

Compared to nonanxious children, anxious children are more inclined to believe that they have little control over external events and circumstances (Chorpita & Barlow, 1998; Weems, Silverman, Rapee, & Pina, 2003) and are less confident in their abilities to perform stressful tasks (Kortlander, Kendall, & Panichelli-Mindel, 1997).

How Do Adults Typically Respond to an Anxious Child?

Parents of anxious children are more likely than parents of nonanxious children to expect their children to be more upset and to be distressed and less competent in the face of challenges. Although this view is understandable given the difficulties that their children are facing, it could lead to parents stepping in and helping more than is actually needed. In support of this suggestion, Creswell, O'Connor, and Brewin (2008) showed that when parents were told that their child might struggle with a puzzle task, they were more involved during the task compared to parents who were told that their child would find it fun (despite the children not differing on how they found the task). Similarly, Hudson et al. (2009) observed that mothers of nonanxious children became more involved when interacting with an anxious child compared to when they interacted with their nonanxious child. Clearly, having an anxious child may encourage parents to respond to their child in a more involved way.

Why Do Anxious Children Need to Be More Independent?

Stepping in and completing a task for an anxious child may reinforce the notion that the child can't cope on his or her own, potentially exacerbating the child's anxiety and maintaining his or her difficulties (Wood, McLeod, Sigman, Hwang, & Chu, 2003; Hudson & Rapee, 2004; Capps, Sigman, Sena, Heoker, & Whalen, 1996). Indeed, when we trained mothers to be more involved in their children's preparations to give a presentation, the children displayed more anxious behaviors when they then had to give the presentation, particularly those children with higher levels of trait anxiety (Thirlwall & Creswell, 2010). Furthermore, it has been suggested that if parents of anxious children engage in unnecessary assistance during relatively nonemotive contexts, their children may find any novel situations to be highly stressful when their parents are not present (Wood et al., 2003). In other words, anxious children may become overly reliant on others, which may lead them to become more anxious when faced with a novel challenge. Helping children to become more independent and to feel more able to take control of their day-to-day lives not only has the potential to increase their confidence and sense of self-efficacy, but also gives parents an opportunity to practice strategies that they will need to help their children overcome fears in a less emotive setting.

What Are the Goals?

- To help parents promote their child's sense of accomplishment and skills in dealing with challenges by increasing the child's level of independence.
- To provide an opportunity for parents to reevaluate their child's capabilities.
- To give parents helpful strategies that will lay the groundwork for helping their child to attempt to face his or her fears as treatment progresses.

How to Do It

Increasing Levels of Independence

It is important to provide parents with a simplified version of the evidence presented above before discussing whether they feel that their child's level of independence is appropriate for their age. If a parent is unsure about whether or not his or her child displays appropriate levels of independence, it can be useful to ask the parent to consider what other children, such as friends or siblings, were doing for themselves at the same age.

Table 4.1 gives some indication of the kinds of daily living activities in which children commonly engage independently at different ages. It can be useful to provide some of the examples from the table during your discussion in order to identify whether there are potential tasks that the child could try on his or her own. Of course, it is important to keep in mind different contexts that may impact on whether or not these tasks are appropriate.

Sticking Points

"When we talked about his level of independence, his parents told me that he already does a lot of things for himself."

Some children might already be relatively independent, and that is great. When this is the case, increasing independence may be less of a focus for intervention. It is important to remember that this can be subjective, however, and that it is rarely the case that there is no opportunity for a child to try something new. We would recommend that every family puts something in place for the child to work on and experience success and thereby boost his or her confidence and sense of achievement in preparation for future work.

"They already try to get their son to do a lot of things for himself, but he gets really upset and it just makes his anxiety worse."

Although it is to be expected that some anxious children find certain tasks hard to do by themselves initially, if the tasks are age-appropriate and the children are given adequate support, then we would expect them to be able to gain a sense of achievement rather than become distressed. If this is not the case, then it may be that the tasks are inappropriate, not interesting and engaging, or simply too hard for that particular child. In these circumstances parents should be encouraged to consider the following questions:

1. Is this the right task to work on to help my child develop a sense of independence?
2. How can my child be motivated to give the task a try (e.g., through making it more engaging or working toward rewards)?
3. How can my child develop the necessary skills to do the task independently (e.g., breaking the task down in to a series of manageable activities and starting with activities that the child has already mastered independently)?

TABLE 4.1. Examples of Age-Appropriate Tasks

Child's developmental stage	Tasks he or she could be doing independently
6–7 years	• Brush teeth • Brush own hair • Set table • Tidy own bedroom • Bring in the newspaper/collect mail from communal area • Vacuum family room • Feed pets • Put on coat and shoes
8–10 years	All the above, plus: • Take out the trash • Water plants • Care for own vegetable garden • Make a purchase in a store • Prepare a simple meal • Wake up with alarm clock • Make bed
11–12 years	All the above, plus: • Take personal care of belongings • Take short trip on public transport • Plan where family will go on a day out • Look up some information for parents on the Internet

For example, the proximity of local stores will determine whether or not the child would be expected to go to them alone.

Identifying Potential Tasks

Try to help parents identify three tasks that they would be happy for their child to try and do independently over the following week. Occasionally parents may suggest things like "washing the dishes" or "washing the car." These suggestions may be perfectly appropriate, but it is important to emphasize that the idea is to try and help children increase their sense of control over their own belongings and well-being. It is important that the child does not see this task as a punishment, but rather as a sign that others feel that he or she is grown-up and competent enough to do more things for him- or herself.

Anxious children will inevitably find some things particularly hard to face on their own, so a good place to start building confidence is to think about areas where they may have already expressed an interest in trying things for themselves or may already occasionally do these things on their own.

Useful Question to Ask Parents

> ➤ "Are there any things that your child is capable of doing, but perhaps at the moment still goes to you for help with?"

Setting Up Success

Despite all the best intentions, children who are used to having help may initially resist doing certain tasks on their own. This can be frustrating for parents as well as making them doubt whether or not their child is actually ready to be more independent. If time is spent preparing parents for this possibility beforehand, they are much better equipped to deal with these setbacks. As such, it is important to talk through the following tips with parents and review them if they encounter difficulties.

• *Show confidence in your child.* Once parents have decided upon the skills or activities they think their child could do on his or her own, it is important that they step back and let their child attempt it. For some parents, this will require effort to tolerate their child's display of some level of negative emotion or distress before stepping in to help him or her. Even if the child doesn't manage the tasks entirely right the first time or becomes a bit upset, parents can tell the child that they are confident that he or she will be able to do it by him- or herself with more practice and then praise the child for having a go.

• *Show the child what is needed beforehand.* If the child has never tried the skill on his or her own before, the parent should talk through the steps required and ask the child if he or she has any questions before getting started. After showing or explaining to the child how to do something, the parent should tell the child that the child is ready to have a go by him- or herself. Once the child has attempted the tasks, the parent should check whether the child has any further questions and answer these before encouraging the child to try it again.

- **Special privileges.** A small reward or special privilege is a nice way to celebrate the child's step toward being more grown-up. For example, if the child is able to wash his or her hair without help, he or she may be able to watch an extra 15 minutes of TV before bedtime.

- **Encourage and stay calm.** If the child struggles and becomes upset, it is important for the parent to stay calm and show that it is OK not to be perfect. Parents should acknowledge their child's feelings and convey that it is to be expected for something to be difficult at first, but that with practice, the child will find it easier.

- **Build up slowly.** If the child shows a lot of distress and finds the task very difficult, the parent should try to break down the task in to parts that the child can do without help and parts with which the parent can help. The parent should gradually cut down the amount of help provided and continue to convey the message that the child will be able to complete the task independently with practice.

- **Give choices.** If the child is very resistant to having a go at something independently, it is important that the parent remains firm in expressing confidence that the child will be able to complete the task without help. However, it can be beneficial to present choices to the child about when or how he or she would like to try the task. For example, if the child is resistant to making his or her own packed lunch, the parent could ask, "Would you like to make a cheese or a ham sandwich?" rather than "Would you like to make a sandwich?" This gives the child a sense of control but doesn't allow him or her to opt out. Equally, giving choices ensures that the parent is happy with the decision that the child makes; for example, making sure that the child makes a sandwich with a filling that the parent is happy for the child to eat.

- **Remain solution-focused.** Sometimes a child can become overwhelmed by the task at hand. If this is the case, parents should share their own experiences of learning a new skill (e.g., "When I learned to do x, I found it useful to do y") and encourage the child to come up with a solution (e.g., "What could you try to do to make this easier?"). Helping parents to get their child to problem-solve is covered in more detail in Chapter 7.

Reflecting on the Child's Coping

By helping the child to become more independent, a parent's beliefs about the child's ability to cope with challenges may also change, making it easier for the parent to continue to promote the child's autonomy. As such, parents should be encouraged to reflect on their child's progress in managing to perform the identified tasks for him- or herself. In particular, it is helpful to ask parents whether they have noticed a difference in their child's level of confidence and whether it has made them think any differently about the sorts of things their child may be able to do independently. Whereas some parents may be surprised by their child's capabilities, others may have expected their child to do these tasks before, but struggled to know how to help him or her achieve these skills. For some families, remaining calm and breaking things down may have been helpful, whereas for others stepping back and showing confidence in their child was the key to success. It is vital that you remain genuinely open and curious as to what works for each family. Whatever has worked for the family is likely to be just as useful when it comes to helping the child face more anxiety-provoking activities going forward.

Useful Questions to Ask Parents

> "What are some things that [the child] now does independently that he or she wasn't doing for him- or herself before?"

> "Have you noticed a change in [the child's] confidence? Has it made a difference to how he or she feels about him- or herself?"

> "Have you been surprised by [the child's] ability to do [insert skill]?"

> "What do you think made it possible for [the child] to develop this skill?"

Encouraging Coping with Worries Independently

Another difficulty for many anxious children is the amount of time they spend worrying. For some, worrisome thoughts can feel as though they are taking over and these children may seek constant reassurance from others. Although it can be tempting to respond by telling a child that he or she does not need to worry, this predictable reassurance can lead to dependence on others and prevent the child from learning to manage worries independently. Instead, if a child seems to be coming to his or her parents repeatedly with worries, it will be important for the parents to help the child develop ways in which the child can control his or her worries without help from others.

Worry Box and Worry Time

In this strategy the child keeps a notebook in which he or she jots down his or her worries throughout the day (or asks someone to jot down the worries if the child is not able). These notes are then put in to a "Worry Box" to be reviewed at a set time—"Worry Time." At the agreed time, parents sit with their child for a set amount of time (limited to roughly half an hour or less for younger children) to talk through the worries together. This can be a useful strategy because it provides parents with an alternative response to reassurance while not dismissing the child's worries; it shows the child that the worry will be listened to but also encourages the child to learn to put the worry aside for a temporary period—providing the child with an opportunity to notice that he or she can indeed control these worries. Furthermore, when the worries are later reviewed, it will sometimes be the case that the child is no longer concerned about a particular worry—thereby providing an opportunity to learn that nothing disastrous happens when worries are not discussed immediately, and that sometimes worries reflect how we feel at that time rather than necessarily reflecting major problems. Parents can use the strategies described in this book (Chapters 5 and 7) to talk through their child's worries in a way that promotes independence.

Some children become really engaged with this process and may create something like a special mailbox that can be decorated however they like. It is important that parents choose a time when they will be able focus all their attention on their child and talk about his or her concerns. This can be challenging if juggling the demands of other children and commitments, so it is important to consider the possible obstacles and to problem-solve with the parent if necessary. It also needs to be at a time when the child will be able to engage in the process (i.e., not when the child is overly tired, hungry, or distracted) and ideally not immediately before bed when the child may be more prone to worrisome thoughts. If a child finds it difficult to wait to discuss his or her worries, it may be useful for the parent to gradually increase the time the child needs to wait to discuss the worry—for example, starting with a few Worry Times within a single day and gradually reducing to less than once a day.

Promoting "Have a Go" Behavior

In addition to helping the child to become more independent, parents should also be given strategies on how to promote "have a go" behavior in feared situations in preparation for future work (see Chapter 6). In order for the child to overcome his or her fears, parents will need to first help the child try things that he or she may be initially scared to do. In order to make this task less daunting for the child, there are some simple but effective ways in which parents can begin to encourage their child to try things he or she typically fears. These include (1) noticing and celebrating bravery (e.g., praising the child), (2) rewarding brave behavior (e.g., extra videogame time) and (3) modeling brave behavior. Each of these is discussed below. Providing parents with sufficient information, including a rationale, will help them share these strategies with others and to make a start on these at home. It is important to review how they have got on with this "encouragement assignment" in future sessions and to recap when necessary.

Noticing and Celebrating Bravery

Due to the nature of the child's difficulties, much parental attention will inevitably have been given to times when their child did not manage to face a fear. Now, in order to help their child draw on inner resources and gain confidence in approaching challenging situations, parents need to watch for and praise their child whenever he or she manages to have a go at doing something challenging. This can be hard because parents will need to notice and praise their child for engaging in behaviors that might be taken for granted in another child. For example, attending a weekend sports club may be a regular occurrence for many children, but would be an achievement for a child who is fearful of interacting with unfamiliar peers and who typically avoids novel social situations.

Useful Questions to Ask Parents

> "Is there anything your child currently does or has tried, despite it being an effort or challenge for him or her?"

> "How could you show your child that you noticed that he or she had a go at something that was hard to do?"

In order for the praise to appear genuine and for the child to feel good about his or her achievement, the praise should be given for a specific behavior and focus on that *behavior* rather than on the child as a person. For example, instead of saying "You were very good today," the parent could say "Earlier when I dropped you off at football, I thought it was great how you went and sat with the other children and waved to me across the car park."

Rewarding Brave Behavior

Another way of giving a child attention for being brave is to use rewards. These could be agreed upon before the child attempts something as a way to encourage motivation. It is also a good fit to pair praise with a predetermined reward. Rewards do not need to be expensive or cost money at all, but they should fit with the achievement the child has made. Ideally a reward should be given whenever the child tries to do something despite feeling apprehensive about it, regardless of the outcome—that is, whether or not they feel different about it afterward. Once a child is given a reward, it is important that it is not removed as a punishment for a later behavior. If this happens, it can discourage the child from engaging in the positive behavior that earned him or her the reward in the first place.

 Sticking Points

"I don't think her parents agree with using rewards; they didn't seem very keen on the idea."

Some parents are unsure about using rewards to celebrate their child's achievements so it is important to check out with parents if this is the case and, if so, to understand why they have reservations and try to answer any concerns that they may have. Below is a list of common reasons that parents give for being unsure about rewards and how we would respond.

- *"Rewards seem like bribery."* If a reward is used as a way of manipulating the child to do what you want then this does seem like bribery. However, we advocate using rewards in order to encourage a child to do something that benefits *them*. It is about celebrating their achievement and showing appreciation for the effort they have put in to attaining a goal.
- *"I can't reward forever."* Rewards are only needed when the child is struggling; once they have overcome a challenge, there is no need to reward. The attainment of their goal becomes the reward.
- *"It seems unfair on my other children."* There may be things that the parent's other children can also work towards during this time. Perhaps this is an opportunity for them to also achieve a goal and receive a reward.

- *"Why reward normal behavior?"* The reward is for the effort the child has made to overcome their struggle. Although the behavior may be 'normal' for others, if it presents a challenge for this child then it is important to acknowledge this and the effort they have made to overcome this challenge.

- *"I can't afford rewards."* Rewards do not need to be expensive. Often children find family activities such as going for a walk, playing a game or cooking a meal together equally or even more special and rewarding. It is important that parents understand the rationale behind giving rewards. They are a way of celebrating and acknowledging that their child has tried/succeeded in doing something that was previously difficult for them. If this is explained to siblings, they can be supportive. If another child is likely to become upset, however, parents could consider whether there are other goals that their sibling could work towards and offer them similar praise and rewards when they have achieved their targets.

Modeling Brave Behavior

Children often learn about the world and what is dangerous by watching and listening to other people. If they see or hear their parents become frightened by something, then it is natural for children to experience the "something" as a genuine threat. However, they can also learn how to cope with fears by watching how their parents and others manage difficulties. Rather than pretending that they never encounter difficulties, parents can identify an area that makes them feel anxious that is appropriate to share with their child and model how to be brave despite feeling nervous or apprehensive. This approach not only teaches a child how to manage anxieties, but also lets the child know that these feelings are normal and that he or she is not the only one who has them. Of course, parents need to consider what are appropriate fears to share with their child (e.g., worries about relationships or money would not be suitable), and they would need to make sure that they are indeed modeling useful coping strategies (i.e., not avoiding the fear).

Useful Questions to Ask Parents

> ➤ "What opportunities might arise in the future where you could show your child that you are being brave?"

> ➤ "Do you or someone close to your child have any fears or worries that you/the other person has had to confront? Would it be OK for your child to know this? How could you show your child how you/the other person overcome these fears?"

Case Example and Therapy Highlights

Eight-year-old Sofia lives with her parents and 13-year-old brother, George. She has always been clingy toward both parents, in particular her mom, but this has worsened since she started school. She is due to go on a camping trip at the end of the year, but her parents are worried about how she will cope. In particular, they don't think she will be able to sleep on her own.

At home, one of her parents must remain upstairs until she is asleep. If she cannot hear them, she calls out for them until one of them responds. Sofia also gets very upset if her parents try to leave her with a babysitter or her grandmother. They have thus avoided going out without her unless it is absolutely necessary. They both agreed that this was putting a strain on their relationship.

Sofia is generally reluctant to spend any time alone. She does not play in her bedroom by herself and does her homework on the kitchen table while her mother prepares dinner. Sofia doesn't report feeling worried about anything, but says she just likes to have company. She does, however, ask her parents to check her homework each evening, and her parents are concerned that she does not understand her schoolwork.

Sofia admits that she finds school difficult. She has made friends, but says she misses her mom. She does not like her teacher and doesn't dare to ask for help at school because, she says, her teacher shouts a lot.

Sofia's mother says that Sofia has always been a sensitive child. She described her as a clingy baby who did not want to be held by anyone but her parents. Although she enjoyed toddler groups and having other children to play with, she always needed her mom close by.

In terms of family background, Sofia and her family have regular contact with her maternal grandmother who lives locally, and Sofia used to stay over at her house quite a lot when she was younger. Although she will visit her grandmother with her brother, Sofia will not stay the night with her unless her mom is there too. Her paternal grandparents live some distance away and thus the family only sees them periodically.

Sofia's father noted that he was quite anxious as a child and that he does still worry excessively from time to time, usually about work-related issues. Sofia's mother said that she is prone to low mood at times and also worries sometimes, particularly about her children.

Promoting Independence

In order for Sofia and her parents to feel less worried about her trip away, she needed to practice feeling more confident when separated from her parents. Although one of the biggest barriers to her going away was her not being able to go to sleep on her own, the therapist suspected that there were also other areas where Sofia could develop skills in becoming less dependent on her parents. Sofia's desire to be with her mother limited her opportunities to experience mastery, and her parents were also uncertain of her capabilities. It was evident from talking to the parents that they both cared for Sofia very much and had sacrificed a lot in order to reduce her distress. They took turns staying with Sofia at night until she fell asleep, and they no longer went out on their own as a couple. The therapist was able to use these examples to commend both parents on their efforts, but it also became apparent that their always being available for Sofia was not helping her to develop confidence.

Sofia's mother initially thought that her daughter's level of independence was right for her age. Although she noticed that other children Sofia's age were perhaps doing more than Sofia, she believed that her daughter needed more help than others and would become upset if she needed to do things on her own. When Sofia's mother spoke about the types of tasks that she helps Sofia with, it seemed to the therapist that she was describing a much younger child. For example, Sofia's mother helped her to brush her teeth, run her bath, and put out her clothes each morning. The therapist acknowledged that Sofia was clearly a sensitive child and that she may need more encouragement than other children her age to practice daily self-help skills for herself.

The therapist discussed how to set up possible tasks with Sofia. Her mother thought that showing Sofia exactly what was needed beforehand would be useful. As a family, they agreed that Sofia should try to get ready for bed on her own. Sofia's goals were to practice brushing her teeth, washing, and getting changed into her pajamas by herself. To her parents' surprise, after three nights, Sofia took this further and also put her dirty clothes in the hamper and laid out fresh clothes for herself.

Her parents liked the use of rewards and decided to celebrate Sofia's new levels of independence by going out for a family meal. Her mother saw an opportunity for Sofia to further develop her skills by encouraging her to order her meal for herself, and despite her mother not agreeing with her choice, she let Sofia make her own decision about what to eat.

The therapist praised Sofia's mother for her response and asked Sofia's parents about whether or not they had noticed any changes in their daughter. Although at this stage she remained unwilling to let her parents go out in the evening, Sofia seemed to have grown in confidence and she also seemed to be very proud of herself. After the first 2 nights her mother had not needed to show her what to do. Seeing their daughter become more outgoing at home made the parents feel more confident about addressing her worries in the future too. They had discussed how they could get Sofia to do more things without them and believed that now she would be more able to cope on a night away from them, compared to previously.

TAKE-HOME MESSAGES

✓ Anxious children may seem more reluctant and less able to do things for themselves compared to nonanxious children.

✓ Parents and other adults may try to step in and help anxious children when they show sign of distress or if they think they won't be able to cope independently.

✓ To feel more confident, anxious children need to be supported in doing things for themselves.

✓ Parents can help by increasing their child's level of independence and promoting "have a go" behavior through praise and rewards as well as by modeling brave behavior themselves.

CHAPTER 5

Helping Parents
to Promote Flexible Thinking
and a "Have a Go" Attitude

Understandably, parents of anxious children will have often tried to help them think differently about their fears by trying to reassure them—for example, saying "Nothing bad is going to happen" or "You'll be absolutely fine"—or putting steps in place to minimize the likelihood of any danger occurring. Unfortunately, despite these efforts, it is not always possible to *persuade* an anxious child to be less anxious. Although there can be short-term benefits from using these strategies, if children only enter a potentially challenging/threatening situation once they feel that all risk has been removed (i.e., either after they have been told there is nothing to worry about or steps have been taken to eliminate any possible danger), they miss the opportunity to learn that they could potentially have coped with the feared situation. Consequently, the initial worry (e.g., "This is going to be terrible") has not been directly challenged by their experiences. Instead, as is discussed in the next chapter, children need to have the opportunity to face their fears if they are to learn something new about both themselves and the situations they fear.

Helping children to face their fears and put them to the test is not an easy feat. However, children can be helped to develop flexible ways of thinking and to become more open to alternative possibilities. In essence, children need to develop what we call "have a go thinking," which is characterized by an ability to consider a broad range of possible outcomes and be curious about the different possibilities, ultimately to promote a willingness to have a go at putting fears to the test. Parents can help children develop "have a go thinking" by asking questions that encourage them to consider that thoughts are just thoughts (i.e., not proven facts) and that there may be different possible outcomes in a feared situation. Although this sounds simple, it can often be challenging, because our natural responses as parents are often to try to convince children that negative outcomes won't occur and that they will be fine. As such, we work with parents to promote an understanding of the rationale for "asking questions rather than giving answers" and to give them an opportunity to practice this approach within sessions.

What the Evidence Tells Us

Do Anxious Children Think Differently from Nonanxious Children?

Cognitive-behavioral theories propose that anxious children become distressed by and avoid certain things because their thoughts are focused on threat and danger. However, it is unclear whether anxious children view things in a more threatening way than nonanxious children. Some studies have found that children with anxiety disorders are more likely than nonanxious children to interpret ambiguous situations in a threatening way (e.g., Alkozei et al., 2014; Waters, Wharton, et al., 2008), whereas others have not found this difference (Creswell et al., 2014; Waters, Craske, et al., 2008; Waite et al., 2015). In a recent study we found that 7- to 10-year-old children appear to be more inclined to focus on threat compared to teenagers (13–16 years old) (Waite et al., 2015), whether they are anxious or not. Instead, what discriminates highly anxious from nonanxious children may be how they *respond* to perceived threat—for example, due to lower confidence in how they would cope with potential threat (e.g., Alfano et al., 2002; Creswell & O'Connor 2011; Waters, Craske, et al., 2008).

Does Treatment Need to Try and Target Negative Thoughts Directly?

Cognitive-behavioral treatment for childhood anxiety disorders typically aims to help children identify threat-focused thoughts and to reevaluate those thoughts by developing more balanced or helpful thoughts regarding the feared situation. However, engaging in these cognitive techniques may not be necessary to help children overcome their anxiety disorder. For example, a recent review concluded that treatments that included both cognitive- and exposure-based strategies and those that focused on exposure only both met criteria for "best supported/well-established treatment" status for childhood anxiety disorders (Higa-McMillan, Francis, Rith-Najarian, & Chorpita, 2015). Furthermore, improvements in self-reported negative thinking have been found to slow down (rather than increase) following the introduction of cognitive restructuring to treatment for childhood anxiety disorders (Peris et al., 2015). Consistent with this research, changes in perceived coping, but not in negative thinking styles, accounted for how much children improved following CBT for child anxiety disorders (Kendall et al., 2016). In relation to guided parent-delivered treatment specifically, there is also a lack of evidence that shifts in children's interpretations and expectations are associated with recovery from anxiety disorders (Thirlwall et al., 2016).

On the basis of the evidence summarized above, it may well be unnecessary for parents to explicitly target their child's threat-focused thoughts and engage in talking-based methods to try to alter them. Instead, there is evidence that the exposure element of treatment may be more critical, particularly for preadolescent children (e.g., Peris et al., 2015). However, because encouraging children to face their fears is difficult, helping them to develop "have a go thinking" can be strategically useful in nudging them to contemplate putting their fears to the test.

What Are the Goals?

- To help parents identify their children's expectations about what will happen when they face their fears.
- To give parents strategies with which to help their children become more flexible in their thinking and to consider alternative perspectives.
- To help parents to encourage their children to test out their fears.
- To give parents opportunities to practice new strategies.

How to Do It

The Role of Negative Expectations

It is important to revisit with parents the notion that how we feel and what we do are often linked to our expectations about what will happen in a given situation. Although it appears that most children may be inclined to see the world in a somewhat threatening way, children who experience difficulties with anxiety may be particularly inhibited and anticipate that they won't be able to cope with the challenge. Parents can be helped to reflect on this point by using Handout 3.1 (in Chapter 3, p. 64).

Identifying Negative Expectations

Whereas some parents are very aware of what their child is expecting to happen in particular situations, other parents may not be sure. This uncertainty is often understandable. When a child becomes very distressed, for example, the parent's focus often fixates on getting through that challenging situation. Then, once it has passed or been managed, the parent may not want to talk about it through fear that doing so may cause further distress

---

 Sticking Point

The child doesn't want to talk to her parents. She gets defensive or says "I don't know" a lot when her parents ask about her worries.

Some children (particularly older children or those approaching adolescence) are uncomfortable talking about their worries with their parents. This can be made worse if parents respond to their child's fears by telling the child why he or she shouldn't think those things (e.g., "Don't be silly—there's nothing to worry about"). Although generally intended as helpful, this response may not only undermine the child's confidence but also make the child less likely to want to share his or her thoughts in future. As discussed, it is important that parents remain genuinely curious and refrain from directly challenging the worries that their child expresses. If a child says "I don't know" a lot, the parents can ask specific questions that require yes/no answers (e.g., "Did John's dog bite you?"). Some parents express concern that introducing worries in this way will make their child worry *more*, but we have not found this to be the case at all. It is also fine for parents to make tentative suggestions (e.g., "Are you worried that the dog is going to bite you?") or, if the child responds well to humor and is not highly distressed, to suggest unlikely (or even a bit ridiculous) things in order to keep the mood lighthearted and for the child to feel that he or she has the upper hand by explaining what is really worrying him or her (e.g., "Are you worried that the dog might run away with your nice shoes?"). Sometimes children do not have a clear sense of why they are frightened in a particular situation. In these cases children can be asked to describe what they think they will do (or not be able to do) in the situation, as it may be this response that they are keen to avoid (e.g., "I don't know what will happen but I will feel really scared and I might cry").

---

or worsen the child's fears. To alleviate these concerns, we share our experience with parents that, although children may find it uncomfortable to talk about their expectations at first, having the opportunity to discuss them with someone who responds helpfully and without passing judgment can be very beneficial. In particular, these discussions can promote understanding about the links between thoughts and feelings, and provide children with the opportunity to consider other possibilities beyond their negative expectations.

Parents who are unsure about what their child is thinking can be given these simple questions to take home and ask their child when their child exhibits fear, worry, or avoidance:

"Why are you worried?"

"What is frightening you?"

"What do you think will happen?"

"What is it about this situation that is making you worried/frightened?"

Although these questions are very simple, the way in which they are asked is critical. In particular, it is essential that they are asked *not* as a challenge (e.g., "What [*on earth*] are you worried about??") but in a nonjudgmental and curious manner.

Cutting Down Reassurance

Offering reassurance is a natural response to a child in distress. However, persistently reassuring the child that he or she has nothing to worry about can potentially prevent the child from assessing the situation independently and learning from his or her experience. It can also make some children feel misunderstood or mistrusting, particularly if they have good reason to believe something bad could happen—for example, if this has happened before or they have heard about it happening to someone else.

Some parents will have recognized their tendency to offer reassurance when their child becomes upset during the earlier discussions about possible maintaining factors (see Chapter 3). If this issue of reassurance has been discussed previously, it is important now to give parents an opportunity to think about whether or not offering reassurance is something they do often and how helpful a strategy it seems to be for their child.

Useful Questions to Ask Parents

➤ "Are there times when you find yourself reassuring your child a lot? Does this help in the short term? And how about the long term?"

➤ "Does your child frequently seek reassurance before trying things? Would your child be able to do *x* without reassurance from you or others?"

Although parents tend to understand the need to cut down their giving of reassurance, it can be an incredibly difficult habit to break, particularly when an anxious child is distressed and asks whether everything will be OK. For this reason, it is important to equip parents with an alternative response. Instead of offering reassurance or their own opinion, parents will need to be supported in learning how to ask the child questions and to help the child to consider other possibilities. Ultimately, the aim is for parents to encourage their child to put his or her expectations to the test and to approach (rather than avoid) the feared situations.

Acknowledging the Child's Expectations and How Those Must Make Him or Her Feel

The first step toward helping children develop "have a go thinking" is to acknowledge their expectations about what will happen and how these must make them feel (e.g., "So you are worried that the other girls won't want to play with you and that makes you feel scared?"). Not only will this articulation help the child feel understood and listened to, but it is also likely to promote the child's understanding of anxiety and the opportunity to label it as such. In addition, this approach promotes acceptance of anxious feelings by conveying the message that "It's OK and understandable that you feel that way." Furthermore, it provides an opportunity to reinforce the message that thoughts are just thoughts, not necessarily facts (see Table 5.1).

Being Curious: Asking the Child Questions Rather Than Giving Answers

Parents can help their children open up to the possibility of being able to learn something new about feared situations by turning reassuring responses to their children's fears and worries into questions that make their children think about other possibilities. This will be a new approach for many

TABLE 5.1. How to Respond to a Child's Negative Expectations

Child negative expectation	Labeling the emotion and accepting the response
"There are monsters in my room."	"That is a very scary thought—I can see why you feel frightened."
"The dog will jump up at me."	"Yes, I can see why thinking that would make you feel nervous about going to the park. It would give you a shock, wouldn't it?"
"Everyone will laugh at me."	"I see, yes, I imagine most people would feel worried about speaking up if they thought everyone would laugh at them."

parents, so it is vital to provide them with examples, such as those outlined in Table 5.2, in order for them to better understand the method.

Useful Questions to Ask Parents

➤ "How would you usually answer your child's question or give him or her reassurance?"

➤ "How could you turn your statement into a question that would help your child think of other possible outcomes?"

TABLE 5.2. How to Turn Reassuring Responses into Questions

Reassuring response	Question to child that conveys curiosity
"Nothing bad will happen."	"What has happened in this situation before?"
"There are no monsters in your room."	"Tell me a bit about what makes you think this?"
"Your teacher will understand if you are late."	"What happens at school when other children are late?"
"That's not going to happen."	"Have those sorts of things happened before?"
	"Tell me about other people who have been in this situation. What happens to them?"
"You'll be fine."	"Have you ever seen this happen to anyone else? What happened then?"

Although children may still believe that something bad will happen, through these discussions they may feel that (1) it's OK for them to feel a bit worried about this situation, but (2) there is some possibility of their feared outcome not occurring (i.e., something bad *might not* happen vs. something bad *will definitely* happen). This addition can represent a helpful shift in the child's thinking toward feeling more confident about "having a go" at testing out his or her fears rather than avoiding them. To manage parents' expectations appropriately, it is important to explain to them that this process is about "sowing the seeds of other possibilities" and building up curiosity rather than convincing their child that nothing bad will happen.

Encouraging the Child to Put Expectations to the Test

Following from this discussion, parents can begin to encourage their child to have a go at putting his or her expectations to the test. Again, it is important that parents don't judge the child's expectations, but instead show curiosity about what could actually happen: for example, by saying "I can see why you would be scared if that did happen. It seems as though there are some other things that could happen too, but it's difficult to know, isn't it?" or "So you said you worry about that happening, and that has happened to someone you know, but sometimes, depending on your teacher's mood, he doesn't shout at all. That's interesting. Sounds like it's a bit difficult to know what would happen if you were late. I wonder which way it would go?"

Putting the child's expectations to the test is discussed further in Chapter 6, which addresses encouraging children to face their fears.

Handout 5.1 provides a useful prompt for parents to take home and complete the above strategies with their child. Share the handout with parents and explain the need to fill it out at home after they have tried this technique with their child, so that you can discuss how it went together in future sessions. It is important to ask parents specifically what questions they asked, how this felt as a process, and how the child responded. Initially, turning reassuring responses into questions can be a difficult skill to master, so it is crucial that parents are given the opportunity to practice with you in a session before implementing it at home. For this reason we devote time to practicing by role-playing scenarios in our sessions. However, once parents are more familiar and comfortable with the technique, they will find that it becomes more natural and, with practice, *being curious* should become part of everyday family conversations. Figure 5.1 shows how a parent might complete Handout 5.1.

Sticking Points

When the parents ask their child to think about other possibilities, the child is stuck because he or she has always avoided the situation and therefore doesn't know what might happen.

In some cases, the child may not have enough information to fully consider possibilities other than the negative outcome he or she is expecting. If this is the case, rather than provide their own ideas, parents can help their child to generate the data needed. This could involve carrying out surveys or observing the situation to see what happens to others. For example, a child who is scared of flying due to the possibility of the airplane crashing, but has never been on a flight, could (1) ask friends and families how many times they have traveled on an airplane and how often they have been in a near crash or actual air accident, or (2) watch planes take off and land at the nearest airport and tally how many crashes he or she witnesses.

The child is too upset to talk about his or her thoughts and engage in these discussions.

There is no hard and fast rule about when parents should have these conversations with their child. Some parents find that they occur most naturally when the child is faced with a difficult situation and is either avoiding it or seeking reassurance. However, some children's level of distress is too high and they are unable to talk about what is worrying them, and/or the parents understandably focus mainly on supporting their child to "just get through it." When this is the case, it is best to wait until the child is calm and to ask these questions in the context of looking back at what had taken place. "Worry Time," which was discussed in Chapter 4, may also be a useful time to hold these conversations.

What is happening?	What is the child thinking? (e.g., Why are you worried?; What do you think will happen?; What is it about [this situation] that is making you worried?)	Acknowledge the child's struggle/Label his or her emotion (e.g., Yes, that would make anyone feel nervous; That must be difficult; Most people would be upset by x too if they thought that; Gosh, that does sound like a frightening thought.)	Ask questions (e.g., What makes you think that [this situation] will happen?; Has that happened to you before?; Have you seen that happen to someone else?; What has happened before [to you/other people])?; What would [someone else] think would happen if he or she was in this situation?)	Promote curiosity (e.g., That's interesting, isn't it?; So, I wonder what would actually happen?; So, it is possible it may happen like that or may not—it's hard to know, I suppose.)
Alex won't go to his grandmother's house.	I asked, "What are you worried about?" Alex said, "She will ask me to clear the table and won't understand." I said, "What is it about that situation that is making you worried?" He said, "If she makes me touch the plates, I'll be sick."	I said that being sick isn't very nice and that most people wouldn't want to be sick either.	I asked, "What has happened before to you?" He got a bit annoyed and I said that I know he's upset because he might be sick. I asked whether it happens to anyone else. He said he doesn't know.	I wondered whether he really would actually be sick if he touched a plate now. Alex wasn't sure. I said that it's hard to know for certain.

FIGURE 5.1. Examples of acknowledging a child's perspective and promoting curiosity.

In-Session Role Play with the Parent

Setting Up and Modeling the Approach

Explain to the parent that you would like to give him or her the opportunity to practice helping his or her child develop other perspectives by going through two role plays in which (1) the parent plays the role of the child and you take the parent role, and (2) you role-play the child and the parent can practice the questions on you/the child. Explain that each role play will last no longer than 10 minutes and that either of you can "press pause" to halt the role play at any point, if either needs to come out of character to think about or discuss anything. Some parents may find role playing to be a daunting task, so it is important to acknowledge that this often can feel a bit funny at first, but that it's a really helpful way to practice before they try it for real with their child.

We think it is most helpful if the therapist plays the role of the parent first because this allows the parent to get a better sense of what is required. It is also a great opportunity for the parent to play the role of his or her child to show you exactly how the child might respond—something that a lot of parents like doing. It is important that the therapist models a "good-enough" example, rather than an outstanding example, to acknowledge that this can be a difficult task and to alleviate any nerves or discomfort the parent may be feeling in trying do this perfectly. Explain to the parent that because he or she knows the child best, it would be good if the parent take the role of the child first and that you will attempt to be the parent. Following the steps outlined in Handout 5.1, confirm that your task as the parent will be to try to identify the child's expectations, acknowledge how these thoughts must make him or her feel, and help the child consider other possibilities. Use information about specific situations that provoke the child to feel anxious that have been collected in previous sessions to focus on in the role play.

Things to Keep in Mind When Playing the Role of the Parent

- Keep your questions simple, following those in the handout as closely as possible so that it is clear to the parent what you are doing. This is not an opportunity to showcase your therapeutic competencies, but to support the parent in learning a new strategy.
- It is OK if you become stuck. You can "press pause" and say that you need a moment to think about the best way to respond. If the parent is doing a good job at playing a "difficult" child, you can acknowledge that it feels hard to know how to respond. Take time to think

collaboratively with the parent about how to proceed in this situation and use this as an opportunity to highlight how useful it is to
practice.

- So as not to overwhelm the parent, don't allow the role play to go on
for too long; stop after 10 minutes or when you think there is enough
material to ask the parent for feedback. If you haven't covered all
three steps, you can talk through together what the next line of questioning may have been.

Feedback after the First Role Play

After the first role play, ask the parent whether he or she thought your
questions (as the parent) would be helpful or unhelpful if posed to his or her
child. Emphasize that you may not have done the exercise perfectly and that
there may be some things that the child would not be responsive to or would
think were silly, and encourage the parent to share his or her thoughts on
what would have been better.

Useful Questions to Ask Parents

> "How did it feel being your child and going through this process?"

> "Were there things I said that were helpful?"

> "Which things might have been unhelpful?"

> "How do you think your child would have responded to the
questions? Do you think he or she would have answered in a
similar way?"

Giving the Parent an Opportunity to Practice

The second role play provides the opportunity for the parent to practice
with the therapist taking the role of the child. Remind the parent that
you can both press pause at any time. Focus the role play on a situation
that is relevant to the child's fears, but try to use a similar scenario to the
one you used in the initial role play so that the parent can easily use this
for guidance. If the parent slips into giving answers instead of remaining
curious and asking questions, pause the role play and offer a possible alternative way of responding, while also picking up on things that the parents
was doing well. Keep a good balance between giving realistic responses
as the child and not making things too difficult for the parent. The aim
is to boost the parent's confidence in trying different ways of responding

to his or her child, as well as ensuring that the parent has understood the technique.

Giving the Parent Feedback

Once the parent has had a go at the role play, it is important to identify and highlight things that he or she did well. We also encourage parents to reflect on the process—in particular, how easy or hard they found it and whether there were particular aspects they thought worked well (or less well). If they slipped into giving answers rather than asking questions, acknowledge how difficult this shift can be, but make sure they have understood the process and reiterate how it becomes easier with practice. Some parents have told us that they have had a go with their partner, which can be a useful way to both practice and share the strategy with other people who care for the child. Of course, if you are conducting the session with both parents, then this is a fantastic opportunity for them to have a go at the role play with one another, after you have demonstrated the technique.

Useful Questions to Ask Parents

➤ "How was it asking questions? Which bits did you think went well? Were there bits you found difficult?"

➤ "Do you think you could do this at home with your child? What would make that easier to do?"

Example of a Role Play: Practicing How to Encourage "Have a Go" Thinking

The following is an example of a role play, using the strategies outlined in Figure 5.1.

> PARENT: Alex, could you please clear the table for me and put the plates in the dishwasher?
>
> THERAPIST (*as child*): No, I can't do it.
>
> PARENT: What are you worried about?
>
> THERAPIST (*as child*): You know what I am worried about.
>
> PARENT: Can you tell me exactly again? I'm struggling a bit and I need you to help me out, so I can understand what you think is going to happen, my love.

THERAPIST (*as child*): Well, I don't want to touch the plates because they are all dirty and I will get all messy, and then I will get sick. That's it.

PARENT: Right, OK. Yes. That is a pretty horrible thought.

THERAPIST (*as child*): Exactly.

PARENT: So what makes you think that's going to happen? Has that happened before when you cleared the plates?

THERAPIST (*as child*): You know I can't bear clearing the plates; it makes me feel really funny, you know that. And then I can't breathe, and it's—ugh, it's terrible.

PARENT: Yes, that does sound horrible. Sorry if I am being really silly here, but I've forgotten, when was the last time that you did this, that that happened?

THERAPIST (*as child*): I don't know. It was a while ago, I haven't cleaned the plates for ages, have I? But you must remember, I did clear them, and I got messy, and, you know, I got really upset.

PARENT: Yes, OK, um. But you just got upset, didn't you? You weren't actually sick.

THERAPIST (*out of role play*): OK, let's press pause quickly. [*Therapist presses pause as the parent slips into giving his or her opinion and giving the child a solution.*]

PARENT: Yes, I know. I couldn't think how to say something in response to that last comment.

THERAPIST (*out of role play*): It is really hard, isn't it? [*Therapist acknowledges the parent's experience.*] But you did a great job of listening to his worries and showing that you understand how that must make him feel. [*Therapist highlights what the parent has done well.*] Well done on that. Do you want to have a quick glance at the handout and maybe try one of those questions? [*Therapist gives the parent an opportunity to think through what might be a good question (rather than providing one) to model promoting independence.*]

PARENT: Yep, OK.

THERAPIST (*out of role play*): Ready?

PARENT: Yes. So you said that you think you'll get sick. Have you seen that happen to someone else?

THERAPIST (*as child*): No. But that's because they don't have my problem.

PARENT: Yes, but if you keep doing it, you will get used to it, and you won't feel so awful, and it will be fine in the end.

THERAPIST (*out of role play*): Let's press pause again. I thought your first question was really useful; it really got me to stop and think. [*Therapist highlights what the parent did well.*] I think you are absolutely right that if he kept doing it, he might not feel so awful. Can you think of any ways that you might be able to turn that into a question so that he could consider a different outcome other than feeling awful? [*Therapist presses pause again since the parent is providing answers. The therapist continues to help the parent to think about possible questions so that he or she feels comfortable asking them at home.*]

PARENT: Um. Maybe I could ask him what would happen if he tried it?

THERAPIST (*out of role play*): That would be a great question, I think. [*Therapist gives encouragement and praise in order to help the parent recognize what he or she has done well to help him or to feel more confident and more likely to try these questions at home.*]

PARENT: So what would happen if you did it more?

THERAPIST (*as child*): I don't know. I'll be sick, I guess.

PARENT: When you were younger, you never got sick. Do you remember?

THERAPIST (*as child*): Yes. [*Although the parent returned to "giving answers" rather than "asking questions," the therapist opted not to interrupt the flow at this point.*]

PARENT: Do you think you might get used to it? [*The parent follows up the previous statement with a helpful question.*]

THERAPIST (*as child*): No. I don't know.

PARENT: Um. OK.

THERAPIST (*out of role play*): Shall we stop there? I thought that was really helpful. I thought you asked some useful questions. Also, I really liked it at the beginning, when you said you were struggling and you needed me to help you understand. [*Therapist reflects on positive aspects of the role play.*]

PARENT: Yeah, when I say things like "Why do you feel like that?," he will close it with "Because I do" or "You know what happens"— and he is right, I *do* know what happens. But saying that I am being a bit silly or have forgotten something, it's making me almost

Sticking Points

It's tough for parents to remember what questions to ask. When we did the role play, it didn't sound very natural.

At the beginning, parents are likely to need quite a bit of practice before this way of responding to their child's worries feels natural to them. Parents might need to explain to their child that they are trying a new approach and might not get it right initially. They can use the Handout 5.1 as a guide and may find it helpful to write out cue cards once they have established useful questions that work best with their child. Through the course of trying the technique, some parents come up with their own question—which is great and to be encouraged. It is quite likely that parents will slip into giving answers from time to time; the main point is that they give their child an opportunity to think for him- or herself about the prospect of other possibilities to what he or she is expecting to happen, to encourage the child to be prepared ultimately to put these fears to the test.

This method is too complicated for the family with which I'm working. It may be OK for parents to do this with older children, but I don't think it's going to work with this particular 7-year-old. She seemed confused by the questions I asked her at the assessment.

What we have described here is much simpler than strategies used in many CBT programs for childhood anxiety disorders, such as using thought records to generate helpful thoughts. Here we are not aiming to get children to draw new conclusions by reflecting on their knowledge and past experience. We are simply starting a process to encourage children to engage in activities that will allow them to learn new things about themselves and their fears. Even if children are not able to think extensively in response to their parents' questions, just the fact that parents are asking questions rather than giving answers is conveying a message that they are curious and that their children's thoughts might need to be put to the test.

be the underdog, so he's not relying on me to sort everything but saying that he's the one who knows his stuff.

THERAPIST (*out of role play*): Yes, that's a really good point. You're not trying to annoy him or anything, you just want to understand his point of view. And often once a young person realizes that you're not trying to convince him or her that he or she is wrong, but that you just want to talk about it and try to help, the young person tends to find these discussions easier. So it is difficult, but I think you did that well. How did it feel for you? [*Therapist asks the parent for feedback and provides an opportunity for reflection.*]

PARENT: Hard not to slip in to getting annoyed by what he way saying. It's hard not to tell him to just do it. But I can see what you're saying; he needs to get to that point.

THERAPIST (*out of role play*): Yes. And in fact, he might be sick again, for all we know. We don't actually know what will happen. But as I said before, we want him to be open to the possibility that maybe he won't, or maybe even if he was, it might not be as bad as before.

PARENT: Hmm. So, yeah, like I always told him it was a one-off, but he does find it disgusting, so he could be sick again, you mean.

THERAPIST (*out of role play*): We don't know. But I think this way of talking with him will help him to think about that a bit more. Do you feel able to practice that, perhaps with another adult at home?

PARENT: I could have a go with Rob.

THERAPIST (*out of role play*): OK, great. Sounds like a great plan to practice first with Rob and then to have a go with Alex and see how it goes. Do you have any questions or comments? [*Ends with an opportunity for questions and further reflection.*]

TAKE-HOME MESSAGES

✓ Parents can encourage their childen to face their fears by helping them to develop curiosity about and flexibility in their thoughts and expectations.

✓ Parents can help their children become more open to "having a go" by acknowledging their children's thoughts and feelings and by asking questions (rather than giving reassurance).

HANDOUT 5.1. Encouraging "Have a Go" Thinking

What is happening?	What is the child thinking? (e.g., Why are you worried?; What do you think will happen?; What is it about [this situation] that is making you worried?)	Acknowledge the child's struggle/Label his or her emotion (e.g., Yes, that would make anyone feel nervous; That must be difficult; Most people would be upset by x too if they thought that; Gosh, that does sound like a frightening thought.)	Ask questions (e.g., What makes you think that [this situation] will happen?; Has that happened to you before?; Have you seen that happen to someone else?; What has happened before [to you/other people])?; What would [someone else] think would happen if he or she was in this situation?)	Promote curiosity (e.g., That's interesting, isn't it?; So, I wonder what would actually happen?; So, it is possible it may happen like that or may not—it's hard to know, I suppose.)

CHAPTER 6

Helping Parents Support Their Child in Facing Fears

Although it is natural for children to want to avoid the things that make them scared, avoidance is a key feature of anxiety difficulties in children (e.g., Kendall, 2012; Barrett et al., 1996). Avoidance has a strong reinforcing quality because it usually results in an immediate significant reduction in aversive anxious feelings. If a child feels bad when he or she is in a particular situation and better when not in that situation, it wouldn't be surprising if the child would rather stay away from that situation altogether. So although avoidance makes perfect sense, and the advantages of reduced anxiety in the short term are very appealing, in the long term avoidance often results in a perpetuation of the fear. Avoidance often means that the child has not been able to disconfirm his or her negative expectations about the feared situation. Through avoidance the child misses out on opportunities to develop coping skills and beliefs about being able to cope with the situation and his or her anxious feelings. For example, if a child who is afraid of spiders has run away from a spider, he or she is likely to continue to think "If I hadn't run out of the room, I wouldn't have been able to deal with it and something awful would have happened!"

The common advice given to someone who is scared of something is to "face your fears." This view is at the heart of exposure therapy for anxiety. The central concept is that in order to overcome fears, individuals need to *expose* themselves to those fears and overcome their avoidance. With the right type of exposure, an individual gets the opportunity to put his or her negative expectations to the test and to experience being able to cope both with the situation and with the resultant anxious feelings. It is important for children to face their fears in a supported way that enables them to learn this new information. Although exposure is a common approach to overcoming anxiety, in practice it is often difficult for children to face up to their fears, and parents understandably find it tricky to know how and when to encourage their children. There are also subtle ways in which children may avoid facing their fears through safety-seeking behaviors. For example, a child may go into an anxiety-provoking situation but engage in reassurance seeking while there, preventing him or her from fully learning about what happens when he or she "faces the fear" completely. In this chapter we outline ways to work with parents so that they can help their children face up to their fears and learn new things about themselves and the situations they fear.

What the Evidence Tells Us

Is Exposure an Effective Intervention for Child Anxiety?

A number of studies have shown that exposure is an effective treatment for anxiety problems (e.g., Hofmann & Smits, 2008; Crawley et al., 2013) and is typically seen as the primary active ingredient of treatments for child anxiety disorders (e.g., Crawley et al., 2013). For example, in multicomponent treatment packages for anxious children, exposure was found to be the key element for achieving anxiety reduction (Kendall et al., 1997; Tiwari, Kendall, Hoff, Harrison, & Fizur, 2013). It has also been suggested that there is typically not enough emphasis on exposure tasks in treatments involving the family and that this area should be a focus of future research (Taboas, McKay, Whiteside, & Storch, 2015).

How Does Exposure Work?

Traditionally, the emphasis in the exposure technique was to work toward habituation and fear reduction in the client (Rachman, 1981; Foa & Kozak, 1986). However, recent studies have demonstrated that outcomes for anxiety treatments are not predicted by either the reported reductions in anxiety levels or by the final anxiety levels during exposure tasks (Craske et al., 2008). Instead, it has been suggested that exposure works through the development of new learning and new memories and the disconfirmation of inaccurate fearful associations (Craske et al., 2008). The authors emphasize that the aim of exposure interventions should not be fear reduction per se, but rather promoting tolerance of the experience of fear. This finding suggests that clients may benefit more from cognitive shifts such as "I did it and coped with it" than from, for example, "My anxiety went down so that means it must be OK." The goal, therefore, is not to make anxiety go away in feared situations but to experience that it is normal and manageable. Hofmann and Smits (2008) also emphasize the point that exposure allows individuals to experience significant shifts in their expectations about the level of harm in feared situations. It's been shown that following exposure tasks, children report higher coping abilities, and that the changes in coping efficacy that occur through treatment are associated with changes in children's anxiety levels (Kendall et al., 2016).

Does Exposure Need to Be Applied in a Specific Way to Achieve the Best Results?

In clinical practice with children, exposure is often applied in a gradual way (e.g., by using a fear hierarchy of tasks that gradually increases in difficulty), but it has been shown that this method is not necessary in order to reduce anxiety—although it does make it more acceptable and manageable for clients (Marks, 1987). This type of graduated approach may be particularly relevant when helping children engage in exposure tasks. Craske et al. (2014) emphasize that exposure tasks should aim to optimize the opportunity for individuals to learn something new about the feared situation. In practice, this may mean that the ultimate exposure tasks need to be broken down in a way that is acceptable and manageable for children and parents, and that the starting point for exposure may be influenced by what the child is prepared to do as a beginning. Practitioners suggest that it is important to spend time evaluating the outcome of exposure tasks to encourage the processing of new learning from the experience. This suggestion is supported by evidence that postevent processing of an exposure task, during which the child's ability to cope with the feared situation is reviewed and emphasized, predicts positive treatment outcomes (Tiwari et al., 2013). Rewarding children for engaging in exposure tasks is also important in promoting engagement and their continued willingness to undergo exposure to feared situations (Bouchard, Mendlowitz, Coles, & Franklin, 2005; Kendall & Ollendick, 2005).

Safety-seeking behaviors are behaviors that help individuals feel safer when encountering anxiety-provoking situations (e.g., phoning Mom several times when not together, seeking frequent verbal reassurance, checking where the toilets are in new places). Research findings are mixed with regard to the use of safety behaviors and the efficacy of exposure. Whereas some research (with adults) suggests that safety-seeking behaviors interfere with exposure by preventing individuals from gaining new information and developing new learning (Foa & Kozac, 1986; Salkovskis, 1991), other evidence suggests that the use of safety behaviors during exposure does not negatively impact the maintenance of fear reduction (e.g., Milosevic & Radomsky, 2008). Few studies have evaluated safety-seeking behaviors in the context of exposure for children with anxiety disorders, although there is some evidence that children with anxiety disorders who use safety-seeking behaviors rather than coping behaviors show a poorer response to treatment (Hedtke, Kendall, & Tiwari, 2009). Ultimately, exposure tasks need to be guided by what the child needs to learn about the situation. Based on current understanding, if safety-seeking behaviors are getting in the way of new learning, then it would be important to encourage the child to engage in exposure tasks without resorting to or relying on his or her safety-seeking behaviors. However, for some children, removing safety behaviors altogether may be a step too far and will leave them resistant to engaging in any exposure tasks. In these circumstances gradual removal of safety-seeking behaviors should be considered as part of the exposure hierarchy (see Sticking Points on page 114).

 Sticking Points

"How on earth do we get parents to do these tasks with their children? Doesn't the child need to do this with a professional?"

This is a concern that we often hear from therapists. There is a preconceived idea that we are the experts in testing out fears and that handing it over to parents may be setting them up to fail. The fact is that parents and children engage in challenging and novel tasks all the time without necessarily giving much thought to it. Parents regularly encounter situations with their children that are unpredictable, anxiety-provoking, surprising, and challenging (e.g., getting stuck in heavy traffic on the way to school on the day of a test). Giving parents specific guidelines on how to set up particular exposure tasks related to usually avoided situations means that we are simply fine-tuning skills that most parents already possess. We are also giving parents permission to encourage their children to approach anxiety-provoking situations—something some parents find very difficult to do without the guidance and "permission" of a professional.

"What if the task goes wrong?"

Of course you need to make sure that tasks will not put the child in any sort of real danger and will not be shaming or damaging in any way. But we can't predict the outcome of all situations and sometimes things do, in fact, go "wrong," as anyone who has put fears to the test in clinical practice will know. The message that we want parents to hold onto is that no matter how the situation transpires during the task, there is always something to be learned and gained from the experience. At the very least, a child can walk away from the task with a helpful interpretation, such as "That went much worse than I thought, but I was OK and I coped with it." In fact, sometimes it is the tasks that go "wrong" that provide the most useful information and opportunity for children to learn about their resilience and their coping abilities. We recall an excellent example of this when a parent was showing her child how to put her hand inside a box with a small spider in it. The spider had some web on it and when the parent took her hand out, the web got stuck to her hand and she accidentally flicked the spider onto the table, right next to the child! This was a lot of exposure at once for that child, and it was a little bit of a shock to begin with. However, once the exposure task was over (and the spider was safely back in its box), the therapist was able to help the child and parent reflect on how well they had both coped with the sudden situation and how harmless the spider had been, even out of its box. You could say the task went a bit "wrong," but in actual fact it had provided a fantastic opportunity for a lot of new learning.

What Are the Goals?

- To help parents understand the rationale for testing out fears with their child in order to:
  - Help their child to change his or her expectations and develop new learning as a result of facing feared situations.
  - Enhance their child's sense of his or her coping ability by confronting his or her own fears and experiencing anxiety.
- To encourage parents to design and implement tasks to test out fears with their child and plan how to apply this strategy.
- To reinforce the importance of using rewards and praise.
- To allow parents to observe and experience their child's reactions and

coping abilities in situations that are normally avoided (which can some-times lead to changes in parents' own expectations and their confidence in their child's ability to cope with challenges).

How to Do It

Giving Parents a Rationale for Facing Fears

It is important that you first give parents a brief rationale for this strategy. Most parents are already familiar with the idea of facing fears, and they may even be able to give you examples of certain fears that their child or other children have already faced and overcome. It's important to give parents the message that facing fears is crucial for their child to overcome anxiety problems. In addition, you need to help parents understand that facing fears helps their child learn whether his or her expectations about the feared situation are accurate. Ultimately, parents need to understand that each new exposure task should create an opportunity for their child to learn something new about the situation and about him- or herself.

Identifying Exposure Tasks

The second task is to encourage parents to come up with ideas for exposure tasks to help their child test his or her fears and to experience being able to cope. The exposure tasks will be driven by the child's expectations about what will happen in a particular situation. For example, if a child predicts that "Mom will get hurt if she goes out in the evenings," ultimately exposure will be focused on the mother going out in the evening. If a child thinks that he or she will feel too horrible when facing a feared situation (e.g., sit-ting near insects), the exposure task will be focused on helping the child experience anxiety in this situation and discover that it is tolerable.

Parents need guidance on how to put the exposure tasks in place with their child. Exposure tasks do not need to be complicated or sophisticated. They simply need to help the child experience a situation that is not nor-mally encountered due to avoidance.

Useful Questions to Ask Parents

➤ "What is your child avoiding because of his or her fears? Is there a situation that your child works very hard to stop from happening because he or she is scared or worried about it?"

> ➤ "We know from the assessment and from our discussions that your child worries the most about *x*? Is there a way we could put this worry to the test through an exposure task?"

The main consideration when planning exposure tasks is to determine what new information the child needs to learn about the given situation and about his or her ability to cope in order to update or change his or her fearful expectations.

We have provided examples below of how a child's fear can be turned into a goal for exposure:

Fearful Expectation	*Exposure Goal*
"Dogs attack and bite people."	Be able to stroke (various) dogs.
"Mom will get hurt if I'm not with her."	Mom goes out in the evening with friends.
"I will be in lots of trouble if my homework is not perfect."	Deliberately make a mistake on homework.
"I will feel embarrassed and won't know what to say if others are listening to me."	Do a short presentation for the class.

 Sticking Point

"The child is too young to be involved in/is not very interested in/is too terrified by the idea to design the hierarchy. How should I suggest that the parents go about it?"

Sometimes parents prefer to plan and apply the steps when it's practical, without too much involvement from the child beforehand, and this can work well with younger children or children who are not very interested in the beginning. Regardless of the approach, it's useful to plan some specific tasks with parents in the session, so that they have a good understanding of the strategy. We also discuss the use of rewards in upcoming material to get children more engaged.

Exposure Using Graded Hierarchies

As discussed above, it is easier for children to accomplish exposure tasks in a graded way due to their understandable reluctance to face their fears. This gradual approach makes it much more manageable for children and often helps engage them in the process. Gradation is accomplished by breaking down the ultimate goal into smaller/easier steps. It's important that each step is closely related to the ultimate goal of the exposure task. We encourage parents to be creative in how they break down the goal into steps and to do this collaboratively with their child. Some children will be able to accomplish the steps more quickly than others, so each graded hierarchy will need to be individually tailored to the given exposure goals, the level of the child's anxiety, and other practical considerations. See Figures 6.1 and 6.2 on pages 112–113 for examples of Molly's graded hierarchies. We have also provided a blank Exposure Plan Form (Handout 6.1) at the end of the chapter for therapists to use with parents.

Useful Questions to Ask Parents

> ➤ "What do you think your child will be prepared to do to start with? Do you think we need to break down this goal into smaller and more manageable steps?"

> ➤ "We want to start with the easiest and work our way to the hardest steps. What do you think should be the order of these steps? Do you think your child will agree with this order?"

 Sticking Point

The parents are worried that their child will be completely put off or daunted by the more challenging tasks and that this may deter the child from the idea of exposure tasks altogether.

If children would be very overwhelmed by the parents' ultimate goal or reluctant for it to happen (e.g., attend school full time), then it can be strategic for parents to start with an "ultimate" goal that is more manageable and appealing for the child (e.g., "be able to go to a friend's to play without parent present"). Parents can then gradually introduce more challenging steps as their child gains confidence in the process.

Introducing the Ideas to Children and Using Rewards

We generally recommend that parents check their ideas for exposure tasks with their child and finalize the graded hierarchies together, in order to involve the child as much as possible and to promote the child's sense of mastery and independence. Parents can introduce exposure tasks to children in a way that encourages them to be curious about the outcomes. For example, explaining that creating exposure tasks is a bit like a scientist in the lab trying to find out new information or to create a new formula. These conversations are also a great opportunity for parents to talk to their child about rewards and to begin to make a plan for how to reward each task. Discuss the use of rewards with parents and emphasize that it's a very important part of helping their child to face his or her fears (see the "Reinforcement of Brave Behavior Using Praise and Rewards," section below, as well as Chapter 4).

In practice what we often find is that parents will implement a graded hierarchy but also encourage "one-off" exposure tasks with their children and take advantage of unplanned opportunities to help their children face fears in various situations as they go about their daily activities. For example, a parent who is helping a socially anxious child may notice an opportunity in the supermarket for the child to go and ask a staff member for help in finding an item. This is perfectly fine and indeed should be encouraged because it helps the child encounter a variety of experiences that will ultimately benefit his or her learning.

Carrying Out the Exposure Tasks

Encourage parents to find out what their child's predictions are before the tasks. Parents can then encourage their child's curiosity about what may actually happen in the situation, as discussed in Chapter 5.

Useful Questions for Parents to Ask Their Children

➤ "What do you think might happen when you try this?"

➤ "What are you worried about?"

➤ "It would be interesting to have a go and see what really happens, wouldn't it?"

It is important that the parent and therapist have a clear plan for what the parent will attempt with his or her child between sessions. It is helpful for

Sticking Point

The child is refusing to go through with the exposure task.

It is helpful to have a discussion with parents about this possibility beforehand. Encourage parents to use rewards to help motivate their child to face fears in these circumstances (see the "Reinforcement of Brave Behavior Using Praise and Rewards" section on page 109 and Chapter 4). Additionally, parents can be prepared to break down the tasks into even smaller steps to help their child accomplish part of the task, rather than avoiding it altogether.

therapists to explicitly discuss with parents when exposure tasks will be carried out and to problem-solve any obstacles that may get in the way of completing the tasks. Sometimes parents are able to do additional tasks, beyond those that have been planned, with their children simply because opportunities for these come up naturally during the course of the week.

Useful Questions to Ask Parents

➤ "When would be the best time to try this exposure task over the next week?"

➤ "Is there anything that's likely to get in the way of this task? How could you overcome this?"

➤ "Sometimes children find the task too difficult when they are faced with it and refuse to go through with it. Can you think of a way of breaking down this task into smaller steps in case your child finds it difficult?"

Making Sense of Outcomes in Relation to Predicted Negative Outcomes and Encouraging New Learning

Once an exposure task has been carried out, it is vital for parents to help their child make sense of the outcome and any new information that has been discovered. This is the time to go back to the earlier predictions and see whether they were correct. These conversations aim to help the child learn from the experience, both about the apparent "dangerousness" of the situation and about his or her own coping abilities.

Useful Questions for Parents to Ask Their Children

➤ "So what happened?"

➤ "Did the predictions/guesses we made earlier come true?"

➤ "What does that mean about [specific situation/you]?"

➤ "What does that tell you about [specific situation/you]?"

➤ "How did it feel?"

➤ "Did you get through it OK?"

➤ "How did you manage to face up to this?"

➤ "How do you feel now?"

➤ "Did you discover anything new?"

➤ "How do you think it will go the next time you are in a similar
   situation?"

Reviewing Progress and Planning Further Exposure Tasks

Encourage parents to review exposure progress regularly and to carry on
planning for more exposure tasks. Children can keep a log of their exposure
tasks, outcomes, and new things they have learned in a "book of exposure
tasks or experiments." This is also a good opportunity to review the outcomes from the parents' points of view and help them think about anything
new that they have learned about their child as a result of the exposure
tasks (e.g., "My child coped much better than I expected"). This review
provides an opportunity for discussing how the parent is likely to respond
to the child in a similar situation in the future (see Chapter 4 for further
discussions about parental responses).

Useful Questions to Ask Parents

➤ "What is the next step on the hierarchy that your child needs to
   accomplish?"

➤ "What else does your child need to learn about this situation?"

➤ "Is there anything that you have discovered about your child from
   this exposure task?"

➤ "How might the outcome of this exposure influence what you do
   or say the next time your child encounters a similar situation?"

Parental Modeling of Facing Fears

There might be opportunities for parents to model facing their own fears (see Chapter 4 for further discussions about parental modeling). This could mean that parents develop ideas for their own exposure tasks and share these with their child when appropriate. Parents could then share their own new learning in different situations with their child. For example, a parent could share with the child a worry about speaking in front of a group of people at work, including his or her anxious predictions about feeling awful and getting words all mixed up, and then the decision to put this fear to the test by volunteering to speak at the next general staff meeting. Once the exposure task is completed, the parent then needs to reflect on what actually happened with his or her child (e.g., "I felt nervous to begin with, but not as awful as I thought I would"; "I did forget to say several things, but on the whole I didn't get my words mixed up—I guess I can handle these things better than I thought").

Reinforcement of Brave Behavior Using Praise and Rewards

Facing up to fears is not easy, and children particularly need help and encouragement to do so. In addition, it is difficult for children to see the longer-term benefits of facing up to things that they usually avoid, so offering a reward can help motivate them to give the challenge a try. Helping parents use rewards with their children was introduced in Chapter 4; providing rewards is a particularly relevant and useful tool when encouraging children to engage in exposure tasks.

Parents need to discuss rewards with their children prior to engaging in specific exposure tasks. Some parents have found it useful to match a list of rewards with a list of exposure steps together with their child. Some children will be very motivated by rewards and will sometimes take on much more ownership of the planning of the exposure tasks to ensure that they earn their rewards.

There are a few important points to remember when using rewards for facing fears:

- Once a reward is chosen and agreed to for a given exposure task, then it must be given following the task as soon as possible.
- If the task for which the reward was selected is not attempted at all, then the reward should not be given (although encouragement to try again is important).

- Sometimes part of a task is completed, and then it is important to reinforce this partial completion in some way. Some parents choose to give the reward for the effort, whereas others prefer to give part of the reward or a smaller reward in this case. This contingency should be planned and agreed to in advance so the child knows what to expect.
- There needs to be a match between the size of the rewards and the difficulty of the tasks so that smaller rewards are given for easier steps and larger rewards are reserved for more difficult tasks.

Rewards do not need to be expensive or fancy. From experience, we have found that children can be very forthcoming with ideas for rewards and often choose rewards that involve time spent doing fun activities, rather than always focusing on material things. See Chapter 4 for further discussion on using rewards.

The following is a list of reward ideas from parents and children with whom we have worked:

- Meaningful praise
- Small candy or chocolate treat
- Football cards
- Chewing gum
- Small doll or animal toy
- Choosing film for family film night
- Favorite meal
- Extra time on the computer/TV
- Points toward a much bigger reward
- Playing together on the computer
- Family board game evening
- Have sleepover
- Trip to the zoo
- New phone app
- Polishing nails together
- Trip to the woods

Case Example and Therapy Highlights

Nine-year-old Molly lives with her mother and father and her younger sister, Eva. The family moved to the countryside recently and Molly has found the move quite difficult. She has become very clingy with her parents, refuses to play with her sister in the large garden, and refuses to go for a walk with the family or to walk to school. Molly's parents have realized that Molly becomes very frightened when she sees animals near the house, especially horses. The house backs onto fields and their neighbors have animals that sometimes come near the back fence of the garden. Molly is also scared of any dark places; she refuses to go to sleep with the lights off and finds it difficult to go into certain places in the house on her own, such as the utility room and the downstairs toilet.

Molly's parents wanted their daughter to overcome her fears of horses and the dark. The therapist helped Molly's parents identify two goals for two separate exposure plans. The first was for Molly to be able to stand near the neighbor's horse and stroke its nose (see Figure 6.1). The second goal for another exposure plan was for Molly to be able to spend 5 minutes in the dark in her bedroom (see Figure 6.2). Although two exposure plans had been identified, the therapist suggested that the parents work on one at a time with Molly so that she did not get overwhelmed. The therapist suggested that the first steps of each plan should be something that are fairly easy for Molly to do so that she can feel a sense of achievement early on. The therapist also emphasized that rewards would be crucial in helping Molly to engage with these tasks and for her to be willing to face up to her fears, particularly because her anxiety in both situations was very high.

Molly first worked her way up on the exposure plan about horses. To everyone's surprise, once Molly completed Step 7 of the first exposure plan, she said she was ready to do Steps 8–10 at the same time. This was an opportunity that Molly's mom did not want to miss, so she encouraged Molly to "go for it." This also meant that Molly received quite a few rewards that afternoon for all her efforts!

The therapist reminded the parents to discuss the outcome of each step with Molly and to help her make sense of any new information that she was learning.

The following is an example of a conversation between Molly and her mother.

MOTHER: I'm proud of you for standing near the back fence today, where you can see the horses. What did you see?

MOLLY: There were two horses there, a brown one and a black one.

MOTHER: What were they doing?

MOLLY: Eating the grass and looking at me sometimes.

MOTHER: Did they run over to you and make loud noises like you thought they would?

MOLLY: No, they looked a bit bored.

Check when completed

Ultimate Goal	To stand next to the neighbor's horse and stroke its nose	
Reward	Trip to see a musical	
Step 9	Hold Mom's hand while she strokes the horse's nose	
Reward	New skirt	
Step 8	Stand next to the neighbor's horse and hold its reins	
Reward	Family games evening; Molly chooses the game	
Step 7	Stand next to the neighbor's horse with Mom holding its reins	
Reward	Make a cake with Mom	
Step 6	Stand a few yards away from the horse but in the same paddock	
Reward	Extra time on the computer	
Step 5	Stand near the back fence of the garden	
Reward	Favorite chocolate bar	
Step 4	Stand near the back fence of the garden with Mom	
Reward	Mom and Molly to go shopping (without Eva)	
Step 3	Spend 10 minutes in the garden on the swings	
Reward	Glitter stickers	
Step 2	Play with sister in the middle of the garden	
Reward	Watch extra half hour of TV on Saturday	
Step 1	Play with sister just outside the back door of the house	
Reward	Lollipop	

FIGURE 6.1. Exposure plan for Molly: Fear of horses.

		Check when completed
Ultimate Goal	To sit in bedroom in the dark for 5 minutes	
Reward	Have a sleepover	
Step 5	Sit in the bedroom in the dark for 2 minutes (take a timer to know when 2 minutes are up)	
Reward	Watch favorite DVD	
Step 4	Spend 30 seconds in bedroom in the dark	
Reward	Go to the park for a picnic	
Step 3	Sit on the stairs with the lights off upstairs for 5 minutes	
Reward	Cupcake from bakery	
Step 2	Spend 5 minutes in the downstairs cloakroom alone, with the lights on	
Reward	Half an hour on Dad's tablet	
Step 1	Walk from room to room in the house and switch the lights off for a moment in each room	
Reward	Magazine	

FIGURE 6.2. Exposure plan for Molly: Fear of darkness.

MOTHER: And how did you feel while you were standing there?

MOLLY: I felt quite nervous because I didn't really know what they were going to do.

MOTHER: But you still did it, didn't you?

MOLLY: Yes.

MOTHER: So what does that tell you then?

MOLLY: Maybe they are used to being around people and they don't really care that I'm there.

MOTHER: And what did it tell you about you?

MOLLY: That I'm really brave.

MOTHER: I think you are! I wonder what else we can find out about horses now that we know you are so brave?

Developmental Considerations

The extent to which children are involved in the planning and reviewing of exposure tasks will depend in some part on their age and abilities. Younger children may find it difficult to make clear predictions prior to exposure tasks, and they may also struggle with developing a clear understanding of the meaning of the outcome of exposure tasks. Once a younger child faces up to a feared situation, parents need to be encouraged to help their child notice that they are coping (e.g., "Well done, that's great that you're

---

 Sticking Points

"The parents have been carrying out the exposure tasks with their child, but it seems that the child is using a lot of safety behaviors in order to cope with each step. Should I tell them to encourage the child to drop these safety behaviors?"

It is advisable to help children to drop their safety-seeking behaviors when:

- They are preventing a child from being able to test out his or her anxious predictions.
- They are getting in the way of the child's being able to tolerate anxious feelings.
- They prevent the child from learning whether he or she can cope in the situation.

Safety-seeking behaviors can be reduced in a gradual way if necessary. For example, a child may be working on facing fears about separation from his or her mom, and the parents have set up steps where the child is spending increasing amounts of time at the grandparents' house, away from the mother. The child is accomplishing these steps by phoning his or her mother several times during each separation. This is helping the child cope with the separation, but ultimately it is also preventing the child from fully engaging in the exposure and being able to test out the prediction that something bad will happen to his or her mother if they are not in contact. In this instance, it would be advisable to introduce a graded hierarchy that reduces the number of times the child phones the mother when separated, aiming toward not phoning at all.

"The child's main worry and prediction is that if he or she doesn't get everything right, he or she will be in trouble or something bad will happen. How can I set up an exposure task to tackle this?"

Ultimately, the child will need to do something less than perfectly in order to learn whether this prediction is right. For obvious reasons, setting up a task that aims for "failure" in some way can be difficult. For example, understandably a parent may not want the child to hand in a piece of homework that isn't to the child's best standard, but doing so could provide an extremely useful learning opportunity that doing work less than perfectly does not result in catastrophic consequences. There may also be other ways in which this could be tested, such as doing his or her hair less than perfectly or by giving an answer in class when he or she is not confident that it is correct.

doing _____! What a brave boy/girl!") and to notice the outcome (e.g., "Wow, what did you think about that? Was it as bad as you thought?").

The way that incentives and rewards are used may be influenced by the child's age and preferences. Younger children respond well to star charts and concrete visual aids to help them see their progress and upcoming reward. In practice, the choice of rewards is usually down to individual preference rather than age; we have come across young teenagers who respond very well to star charts as well! Most children will need to receive the rewards as soon as possible after completing the task in order to enhance the reinforcing quality of the rewards. Older children are better equipped to hold the reward in mind if there is a delay between the task and when the reward is given and might even prefer to "save up" a reward toward a bigger reward.

TAKE-HOME MESSAGES

✓ Exposure is an effective and evidence-based strategy for the reduction of anxiety in children.

✓ The aim of exposure tasks is to help children test their predictions and learn new information about anxiety-provoking situations and about their ability to cope with anxious feelings.

✓ Parents are well placed to carry out exposure tasks with their children in situations that are encountered in daily life.

✓ Giving parents specific guidelines about how to implement exposure tasks with their children will enhance parents' confidence in using this strategy and increase the chances of success.

HANDOUT 6.1. Exposure Plan Form

Check when completed

Ultimate Goal		
Reward		
Step 9		
Reward		
Step 8		
Reward		
Step 7		
Reward		
Step 6		
Reward		

(continued)

Step 5		
Reward		
Step 4		
Reward		
Step 3		
Reward		
Step 2		
Reward		
Step 1		
Reward		

CHAPTER 7

Helping Parents Promote
Independent Problem Solving

Problem solving perhaps doesn't get the credit it deserves when it comes to therapeutic interventions. It is often included in CBT packages but is sometimes overshadowed by other strategies such as thought challenging and exposure. It is also often seen as "common sense" or a skill that should be obvious and instinctive for many. Although it is true that problem solving is a simple and structured skill that is fairly easy to learn, it is often the case that children with anxiety disorders and other mental health problems simply do not apply this strategy on a regular basis. In clinical practice we clearly see that an ability to effectively problem-solve in different situations and in relation to different worries can have a significant positive effect on a child's sense of confidence and mental health in general.

The fact is that many of us problem-solve all of the time. From the minute you wake up and go through your morning routine, you no doubt encounter things that need some degree of problem solving. These may be small things, such as discovering that you have run out of coffee, or quite major things, such as realizing that your car won't start and you need to get the kids to school. Some problems or issues will feel easy to deal with and you may do it automatically, whereas others may feel very tricky and even overwhelming at times. The ability to respond to problems and issues in a helpful and proactive way can make a big difference to our resulting emotional responses. Approaching a problem head-on and tackling it in a systematic and planned way will often mean that a useful solution can be found and the problem can be overcome. Not surprisingly this process may lead to feelings of relief, competence, confidence, calmness, and positivity. Avoiding dealing with things (as discussed in Chapter 6) can have the opposite effect and may lead to stress, worry, anxiety, reduced confidence, and even low mood and low self-esteem in the long run.

We find that anxious children often rely on others to deal with things for them. Although this sounds understandable and acceptable on the surface, it does mean that over time, these children may develop unhelpful beliefs about themselves, such as "I can't cope on my own"; "I need help from others"; "I won't be able to handle things"; "The world is overwhelming"; "Problems are awful"; and so on. With repeated experiences of others always coming to the rescue, a child may eventually have reduced confidence and lower self-esteem, particularly if comparing him- or herself to peers who display more coping and independent behaviors.

Parents can help their child to engage in problem solving more often and more independently. As discussed in Chapter 4, it is important for parents to promote autonomy, and this strategy provides a fairly simple and concrete opportunity for doing so. By encouraging their child to problem-solve, parents can enhance his or her sense of coping ability and skills.

What the Evidence Tells Us

Does Problem Solving Lead to Reduced Anxiety in Children?

Although therapists often observe the usefulness of teaching children problem-solving strategies in clinical practice, there is very little research on the specific relationship between problem solving and anxiety in children. Problem solving is a strategy that is usually embedded within established CBT treatment packages for children with anxiety (e.g., Kendall & Hedtke, 2006; Stallard, 2003; Spence, 1995). Although it has been established that some of these CBT interventions are helpful for a proportion of young people with anxiety (James et al., 2013), the relative contributions of particular specific aspects of the treatment packages, such as problem solving, remain unclear.

Do Children with Anxiety Have Reduced Abilities to Problem-Solve?

The adult literature indicates that anxiety is associated with lower problem-solving confidence but not with actual problem-solving skills (e.g., Davey, 1994; Kant, D'Zurilla & Maydeu-Olivares, 1997; Ladouceur, Blais, Freeston, & Dugas, 1998). Similarly, children who worry excessively also tend to have lower confidence in their problem-solving ability compared with low worriers (Parkinson & Creswell, 2011), despite having similar problem-solving skills. Therefore, it seems that anxious children have the skills in place but lack the confidence to put the skills into practice due to unhelpful beliefs about their abilities. This finding has obvious clinical implications; it may be helpful, for example, to encourage anxious children to engage more in problem solving despite their beliefs and low confidence. It may also be useful to increase children's confidence about using this strategy so that they are more able to apply their problem-solving skills. For example, in one case study, Gallant (2013) targeted problem-solving confidence with a young person and helped her to successfully overcome worry.

Do Anxious Children Have a More Avoidant Style?

In addition to having low problem-solving confidence, children with higher levels of anxiety and worry also appear to be more avoidant in their problem-solving style. Specifically, children who worry more also tend to choose more avoidant solutions to hypothetical social problem-solving situations (Wilson & Hughes, 2011). Furthermore, compared with nonanxious children, anxious children are more likely to choose avoidant responses to ambiguous situations (e.g., Barrett et al., 1996; Waters, Craske, et al., 2008; Waite et al., 2015). These findings suggest that children may become "stuck" at two possible avoidant points in the problem-solving process: firstly, in not having enough confidence to actually implement their problem-solving skills; and secondly, in implementing the strategy in a way that will help them actually face the problem, rather than relying on avoidant solutions that may lead to further anxiety.

It's clear that further research needs to be conducted to guide our decision making about whether and how much problem solving can be helpful for reducing anxiety in children, although the available evidence, as discussed above, provides some useful pointers. We can also be guided by clinical experience and individual formulations to help us implement this strategy appropriately and with good effect.

When to Use Problem Solving

- *When the child is experiencing realistic anxious thoughts and/ or thoughts about things that may happen.* Some anxious thoughts may reflect actual real problems that the child is facing (e.g., "I've had an argument with my best friend and she's not talking to me") or things that *may* happen, even though less likely (e.g., "I'll be told off at school"). Problem solving is a useful strategy for tackling these types of anxious thoughts.

- *When the child is ruminating.* Rumination happens when thoughts turn over and over in the mind, without leading to any resolution. Rumination is associated with a lot of "why" questions, such as "Why has this happened?" or "Why is she doing this to me?" Problem solving helps people move away from rumination, which can often cause anxiety, and move into action. Action is more associated with "how" questions, such as "How can I deal with this?" or "How can I get some help?"

- *When there are obstacles to putting treatment plans in place.* Problem solving can help children and parents overcome obstacles during the treatment program (e.g., the child is prepared to work on answering questions in class, but the teacher never picks him or her).

What Are the Goals?

- To explain to parents the rationale for using problem solving to:
  - Help their child deal with and overcome realistic anxious thoughts and problems more independently.
  - Reduce their child's rumination.
  - Enhance their child's sense of his or her own coping ability.
  - Increase their child's level of confidence and general independence.
- To encourage parents to learn the problem-solving strategy by experiencing the problem-solving process firsthand.
- To help parents plan for the application of the strategy with their children.
- To identify any obstacles to practicing and apply problem solving to overcome these.

How to Do It

Working through This Strategy with the Parents

When presenting this strategy to parents, it is helpful to do so in an experiential way. That is, it is useful to actually go through the problem-solving process with parents using one of their own chosen problems. This approach works well for a number of reasons. Firstly, parents get to experience firsthand what it is like to be guided through a problem-solving process toward a solution. They can therefore have more of an understanding of what this will feel like when they apply the strategy with their child. Secondly, teaching the strategy in this way makes it more interesting and engaging for the parents, which hopefully helps parents remember the main points and motivates them to use it with their child. Thirdly, many parents find the strategy useful for solving their own difficulties, especially when they become stuck on a problem, so going through the process with them in this way aids their all-around problem-solving attempts. It's useful to write down the answers as you're going through the problem-solving process, so that it is easier to remember the main points and go back to at a later point. Ask the parent to do the writing if possible. We have provided a sample problem-solving sheet (see Handout 7.1 at the end of the chapter) for you to use at the end of this chapter; also see an example later in this chapter (p. 131).

Using Common Obstacles Encountered by Parents When Applying the Anxiety Treatment Program

When demonstrating the process with parents, use examples of obstacles that are often encountered by the parents who are working through this program. This is a perfect opportunity to discuss problem solving with parents and to demonstrate the technique in relation to the particular problem they're having.

Figure 7.1 lists some common obstacles that parents may face in helping their child overcome difficulties with anxiety.

Teaching the Strategy

The problem-solving strategy is best taught in a series of structured steps so that it is more explicit and memorable for parents. We have provided an excerpt from a session with Anna, Ryan's mother, in order to demonstrate the type of conversations to have (see pp. 128–133). When going through problem solving with parents, it is important to encourage as much independent thinking as possible and not to get pulled into giving parents answers or ideas. Taking this approach models how you want parents to enact the strategy with their child.

Problem solving involves the following main steps:

- Step 1: Identifying and summarizing the problem
- Step 2: Brainstorming ideas
- Step 3: Evaluating each idea in detail
- Step 4: Choosing the most appropriate solution or solutions
- Step 5: Planning how to implement the chosen solution(s)
- Step 6: Identifying any obstacles
- Step 7: Applying solution(s)
- Step 8: Reviewing the outcome and planning further, if needed

---

Practical problems

- "I don't have enough time to do the exercises."
- "My partner hasn't been able to come to the sessions and he/she is not involved in working on our child's anxiety."
- "It is quicker (easier) to just do something for my child, rather than try to get him/her to do it."
- "I don't know when to push my child. Is he/she anxious or just not interested?"
- "Other family members have different ideas about what is the right thing to do."
- "When my child 'acts up,' I don't know if this is because he/she is upset or being difficult."
- "I'm not there at the times that my child worries about."
- "It seems unfair to my other children to be rewarding one child for doing things they do all the time."
- "We know what our child needs to do to overcome his/her fears, but those situations don't happen very often in everyday life."

Personal problems

- "I find it hard to stay motivated to keep 'pushing' my child."
- "I can't help worrying about how my child will be able to manage if I give him/her a push."
- "It is hard to push my child to do something when there are other members of the family who have the same problem and are not doing anything about it."

FIGURE 7.1. Common problems that parents may face in helping their child overcome difficulties with anxiety.

Step 1: Identifying and Summarizing the Problem

This is an important step that sometimes gets overlooked. If you don't know precisely what the problem is, then it is difficult to move toward finding a solution for it. Vague descriptions of a problem, such as "I'm busy," may lead to vague solutions (e.g., "Do less"). It is much more useful to break down a bigger problem such as this into more concrete and specific parts, and to work on these one by one using the problem-solving approach. For example, the problem that "I'm busy" may be comprised of more specific problems, such as "I need my husband to help more with the children"; "My working hours currently are more than I signed up for"; or "I do too many chores in the house on my own."

A useful way to identify the problem is to ask the parent to describe it in one or two sentences and to say why it is a problem for him or her. Then help the parent to be more specific by summarizing his or her description of the problem and pulling out particular elements. Together, agree which of these specific problems you will work on first.

> ## Useful Questions to Ask Parents
>
> ➤ "How would you summarize what you have just described to me in one or two sentences?"
>
> ➤ "What is it about this situation that makes it a problem for you/ your family?"

Step 2: Brainstorming Ideas

Brainstorming is a crucial step. Generating possible ideas marks the beginning of facing up to the problem and challenges those "It's awful"/"I won't be able to cope" thoughts. It is important to devote enough time to this step so that the parent is able to come up with a good list of ideas. Praise parents for any ideas that they are able to generate. Some people aim to find the "perfect solution" and can get stuck on this goal. Chances are, for most problems, there is no perfect solution, and so it is important not to judge any of the ideas at this stage. Instead, ask parents to write down whatever comes into their heads, no matter how wacky or ridiculous the ideas seem to be at the time. Again, often people will discount their ideas because they think "That will never work" or "That's just never going to happen." This defeatist thinking can get them stuck. Allowing for those weird and wonderful ideas can sometimes free the mind to find other ideas, so it's good to make this part of the process lighthearted, especially when using the technique with children.

The key messages for facilitating this step are (1) to take on board and praise *any* ideas that come up while parents are brainstorming; and (2) to stop parents from starting to evaluate their ideas at this point, because negative judgments can get in the way of their generating further ideas. Often in the beginning, parents can see no solution or only one, but given enough time and encouragement, parents generally start to generate additional ideas.

Step 3: Evaluating Each Idea in Detail

Once all the options have been clearly identified, it is time to evaluate each one in more detail. This is a chance for the parent to think about how feasible each idea is in terms of being able to apply it to the problem and how helpful it will be in resolving the difficulty. Once again, it is helpful to encourage parents to be realistic in their expectations about how "perfect" the solutions need to be. Encourage an approach of "good-enough" and "OK" solutions. Ask parents to rate each solution according to how *good* the expected outcome of each one is and how *doable* it is on a 10-point scale (1–10) (see Handout 7.1). Tell parents to ask their child very specific, focused questions to help their child consider both short- and long-term consequences for each idea (e.g., "What would happen after 1 week if we chose this idea?"; "What about after 1 month?").

Step 4: Choosing the Most Appropriate Solution or Solutions

Now it's time to choose the most helpful/appropriate solution or solutions. As just noted, encourage parents to choose something that is "good enough" to get the ball rolling on tackling the problem. They can choose the best/ easiest to implement solution based on the ratings that they assigned to each one. It's key that therapists let parents come up with their own ideas and their own choices. This is also crucial when parents implement the strategy with their child because it encourages independence and confidence in using the strategy.

Steps 5 and 6: Planning How to Implement the Chosen Solution(s) and Identifying Any Obstacles

Once the best solution has been chosen, encourage the parent to think about and plan for how it will be implemented. Together, you may need to consider factors such as timing, where the parent will implement the solution, whether help from anyone else is needed, and any obstacles that may get in the way and how to overcome these.

Step 7: Applying Solution(s)

Parents then need to have a go at applying the solution between sessions using the plan from Steps 5 and 6.

Step 8: Reviewing Outcomes and Planning Further, If Needed

It is important to review how this process went at the following session. Did the parent follow the problem-solving steps? If not, what got in the way? How can the parent apply the solution next time? If the parent did implement the solution, how did it go? Did it solve the problem? Maybe just a little? What did the parent learn from the process? If the problem is still present, what other solutions can the parent try next? How will the parent put these in place?

Case Example and Therapy Highlights

Ryan, who recently turned 11 years old, worries about many things a lot of the time. His worrying has been getting progressively worse over the past year or so. His mother, Anna, recalled that Ryan had always been a sensitive child and would often ask many questions about various things, especially if he was going to encounter any new situations.

Many of Ryan's current worries revolve around school-related matters as well as the well-being of his family. Ryan particularly worries about his 4-year-old sister, Ellen. He watches her closely when he is out with his mother and Ellen, and sometimes he even tells his mom to watch Ellen more carefully if he thinks she might be in any danger. For example, Ellen loves feeding the ducks at a nearby pond in the park, and this situation makes Ryan extremely anxious because he worries that she will slip and fall into the water. Ryan also worries about his mom and dad, especially if he knows that his dad is going on a long trip for work.

Ryan worries quite a lot about his homework and about remembering to take everything he needs for school every day. He checks his schoolbag many times in the evenings to make sure he hasn't forgotten anything. He also tends to spend a lot of time on his homework and will go over things repeatedly to make sure they are all right. Ryan worries a lot about getting things right, and when he has tests at school he becomes extremely anxious for a few days before and sometimes is unable to sleep for most of the night before the test.

Once Ryan starts worrying about something, it is very difficult for him to stop worrying, even if he is doing something enjoyable. Sometimes when he is very worried, Ryan becomes very snappy and irritable, and at other times, he is tearful and quite low in spirits. When he is worrying about something, his mom tends to spend extra time with Ryan to reassure and help him in various ways. Anna has become involved in helping Ryan feel reassured about his schoolbag and she checks it with him and reminds him that he has everything he needs. Anna also keeps telling Ryan that Ellen is fine and that he has nothing to worry about. Although this reassurance seems to work some of the time to calm him down, it never helps for very long before Ryan quickly reverts to feeling anxious. Anna also tries to remind Ryan that she will be there to help him with anything he needs, even if it is at school. She tells him that she can always come to school and sort things out if he has forgotten anything or if there is any other problem.

Anna admits that she does understand Ryan's tendency to worry because she herself is a bit of a worrier. She tries to hide her worries from Ryan but wonders whether he can tell when she is anxious. She tends to become very quiet and serious when she is worrying a lot about something, and Ryan often asks her if she is OK at these times.

On the positive side, Ryan has a good group of friends at school and gets good grades. He enjoys playing rugby and cricket on the weekends, and he gets on well with his family and grandparents, whom he sees almost every week.

It was clear to the therapist who was working with Anna that Ryan was often making catastrophic predictions that were making it hard for him to face his fears. Using "have a go" thinking (see Chapter 5) to help him face his fears (see Chapter 6) for these types of worries could be very useful for Ryan. It was also clear that some of Ryan's worries were based on things that could indeed happen. For example, it was likely that Ryan would one day forget to bring something important to school, and his school did take a very hard line in this area. It was also very likely that he would not get his homework right every time or pass every single test, and as a result, he might receive some sort of negative feedback. Although these worries hadn't actually happened yet, the fact that they were quite likely to happen at some time meant that they were well suited to a problem-solving approach. The therapist hypothesized that if Ryan had a realistic plan about how to respond in these situations, should they arise, he might feel much less worried about them and instead feel more confident about his coping abilities.

An excerpt from a therapy session with Anna follows.

THERAPIST: Often children worry about things happening that may well actually happen. A good example may be when a child is worrying about being picked on or about getting told off at school. Ryan has his own list of worries, as we know. While it can be useful to encourage Ryan to use have a go thinking [*Reminding the parent about other useful strategies from the program.*] in these situations, it may also be useful to help him think about what he would do if one of the things that worries him did happen. Helping Ryan directly through problem solving is useful because it would help him feel that he can do something about the problem and cope with the situation independently if it happens, and therefore reduce his tendency to feel anxious about it. [*Providing the parent rationale for the strategy.*]

ANNA: Yes, that makes sense. Ryan just thinks that I'm going to sort everything out for him, so I don't really think he ever gets a chance think about it properly himself.

THERAPIST: It's great that he has such high confidence in your ability to support him, and this obviously gives him a lot of comfort. [*Picking up on what the parent is already doing well and praising him or her.*] The tricky thing is that you can't always be there to sort things out for him, and if he relies on your help too much, then he's less likely to feel he can cope himself. [*Returning to rationale.*]

ANNA: I'm the "sorter" in the family. I sort everything out for everyone, and to be honest, it would be nice just to not have to do this all the time, even with my husband.

THERAPIST: Sounds like you deserve a good break from sorting things out for others. [*Acknowledging the parent's situation.*] OK, I want to go through the problem-solving strategy with you in detail so that after the session, you can use it with Ryan and see how he gets on. Is that OK? [*Introducing the strategy and session talk.*]

ANNA: That's fine.

THERAPIST: I find the best way to go through the strategy is to actually help *you* to go through the problem-solving process. Then you can do the same with Ryan and one of his problems. [*Setting up the format of the session task and giving rationale for the approach.*] I have a list here of problems that parents have encountered when trying to implement this treatment program with their children [shows Figure 7.1]. Are any of these relevant for you? [*Showing list of problems other parents have encountered, which can be validating to parents. Identifying the main problem to work on.*]

ANNA: OK, I guess this one here, about getting other family members involved in the treatment program. I'd like my husband, John, to be a bit more involved in helping me to work on Ryan's anxiety.

THERAPIST: That sounds like a really worthwhile issue to think about. Great, let's focus on that. [*Acknowledging the main issue for the parent and encouraging the parent to take the lead on what is being discussed.*] I'm going to talk you through the main steps of problem solving while we focus on your chosen problem. . . . [*Systematically going through the main steps of problem solving with the parent.*] Could you describe in a couple of sentences what the problem is and why it's a problem for you? [*Helping the parent to summarize the main problem.*]

ANNA: Well, I suppose the problem is that I'm doing everything from this program with Ryan, and this leaves me little time for other things that I really need to do. It also means that my husband doesn't really understand the things I'm working on with Ryan's anxiety and he sometimes does the opposite to what I'm trying to achieve.

THERAPIST: Right, sounds like the main problem is not having Ryan's dad on board with the treatment program, which means you do it all and he doesn't fully understand the approaches you're trying out. [*Reflecting back the summary of the main problem to the parent to check accuracy.*]

ANNA: That sounds about right.

THERAPIST: Let's write it down on this worksheet [Figure 7.2]. Are you happy to do the writing? [*Handing over control of the task.*]OK, now that we know what the problem is, let's come up with some things that you can do to try and solve it. [*Encouraging the parent to generate ideas.*]

ANNA: Well, I suppose I could ask John to look at the handouts and read the notes. But that won't work because he gets bored so easily. . . .

THERAPIST: OK, that sounds fine. [*Positively reinforcing the parent's first idea.*] Let's write that idea down and let's hold off with judging it and evaluating whether it will work or not for a bit later on. [*Encouraging an open mind at this point and discouraging evaluation of the idea.*] What other ideas come to your mind? Don't worry if they seem completely unrealistic or unhelpful at first—we just want to get as many ideas down as we can about what you could do. [*Encouraging the parent to brainstorm and come up with other ideas.*]

Now that we have a list of things that you could do, let's think about each one in terms of how good you think it is at solving the problem and how doable it is. We will use this rating system from 0 to 10 to give each solution a rating. . . . [*Helping the parent to systematically evaluate each idea.*] So out of this list of solutions that you have come up with, based on the scores you have provided, which one looks like the best one to try or the one that's most OK compared with the others? [*Encouraging the parent to choose a solution that seems helpful.*]

ANNA: I think, realistically, it's the one about setting some time aside to talk to my husband about the program and then giving him specific things to work on with Ryan.

What is the problem?	What could I do?	What would happen if I did this?	Rating (0–10)	
			How good would this be?	How easy would this be to do?
John is not doing the treatment program, and he doesn't understand the things I'm trying out.	Ask him to read the treatment notes and look at the handouts.	He gets bored easily and has a short attention span, especially when he is tired after work, so he probably wouldn't do it.	5	4
	Give him a summary of the main things that I'm trying out with Ryan.	He might be able to take some of this on board and perhaps take a lead on one or two things.	6	5
	Carry on doing it myself.	This won't solve the problem, although it does feel like the easiest option.	2	8
	Introduce one idea at a time to John and ask him to help with that one thing (e.g., help Ryan face a step on his exposure hierarchy).	This will probably feel like the most manageable thing for John, as he is so busy at work.	9	9
	Forget the whole thing altogether!	Nice thought, but it certainly won't help anyone.	0	10

FIGURE 7.2. Anna's Problem-Solving Worksheet.

THERAPIST: Great. [*Praise.*] So how soon do you want to do this? [*Helping the parent to plan to put the solution into practice.*]

ANNA: Tonight!

THERAPIST: Great. Can you predict any obstacles to getting this started? [*Helping the parent to plan for any difficulties that might get in the way of implementing the solution.*]

ANNA: Only if my husband is home from work too late to be able to discuss it properly with him. If he is late, then I'll wait until Saturday because I know he has nothing on that day.

THERAPIST: That sounds like a good plan. [*Positive reinforcement.*] We can review how everything went the next time we meet. If needed, you can always go back to your list and try some of the other solutions you came up with. [*Introducing flexibility in how the strategy can be used. Giving the message that the use of the strategy will be discussed again at the next session.*]

The therapist then returned to some of Ryan's concerns and encouraged Anna to think about using the problem-solving strategy with Ryan, in the same way that they had just done for her problem.

THERAPIST: Hopefully, going through this strategy together has highlighted its key elements, and now you will know what it will feel like for Ryan when you go through the same process with him. [*Encouraging the parent to reflect on using the strategy with Ryan.*] It's important to let him come up with his own ideas, so only make some small suggestions to get his thinking going if he's completely stuck. It's all about giving him the confidence that he can find solutions to his problems independently, so that he becomes a confident and independent problem solver. [*Giving a clear message about granting autonomy.*] What problems do you think might be worth focusing on with Ryan? [*Helping the parent to start thinking about using the strategy with Ryan.*]

ANNA: Well, following from our earlier discussion, I wonder whether I could help him to think about what he would do if he discovered at school that he had forgotten something important.

THERAPIST: I had the same one in mind. Great, so keep that one up your sleeve. You might also find that Ryan wants to work on another problem altogether when you ask him, so in the beginning I suggest that you let him lead you, so that he feels like he's in charge of the whole process. [*Giving the message that it's good to have something prepared but focusing on letting Ryan take the lead.*] How do you feel about trying this with him over the next week?

ANNA: Fine. I think he will like it because he is a very logical thinker and he likes to write things down. He also likes it when I sit down and talk things through with him.

THERAPIST: I look forward to hearing about how this goes at our next session. [*Giving the message that this is important to try between sessions and the therapist will come back to it next time.*] Do you have any questions or anything you are unsure about in relation to problem solving? [*Checking on any final difficulties or concerns with the parent.*]

ANNA: No, it seems like a straightforward approach. I'll see what Ryan thinks.

Developmental Considerations

With very young children there will be a limit to how much the problem-solving strategy can be covered in detail. It may be that the strategy needs to be simplified with the use of fewer steps—for example, teaching younger children to "stop" when they have a problem, "think" about two or three ideas, and "go" and try them out to see if it helps. Paul Stallard (2005) presents a child-friendly version of a traffic light system for encouraging problem solving in his "Think Good—Feel Good" program.

 Sticking Points

"The parents are finding it difficult to pin down their child to work on problems in a systematic way, and sometimes they find it difficult to pin him down at all to sit and talk through it. What should I advise?"

When children are reluctant to sit down and work through problems on paper with their parent, parents may need to apply the approach in a conversational way. A lot of parents have found it useful to talk through the strategy when in the car with their child (there's no getting away from it in the car!) or to do it "on the go" when out doing other things together (e.g., arriving at sports or ballet class and realizing that something important has been left behind). It can also be useful to suggest a reward system for working on problems together.

*"We haven't covered problem solving yet in the treatment program,
but it seems relevant to some of the obstacles that parents are
coming up against right now. Can I introduce the problem-solving
strategy early on in the treatment program if needed?"*

Some therapists find that problem solving becomes very relevant early
on in the treatment sessions when parents encounter obstacles in working on anxiety with their child. Although we generally advise that this
treatment program be covered with parents in the order that we have
presented it in the book, problem solving can be introduced early on if
needed—and, in fact, it can be very useful in helping parents to engage
with the program and make progress.

*"When reviewing the problem-solving strategy with parents, it is
apparent that they are taking over and noting down all of their own
ideas and consequences. Won't this get in the way of helping their
child to learn to be independent?"*

The key thing to remember is to help both parents and children to
become independent problem solvers. If you notice that the parents are
doing everything, firstly, pick up on things that have gone well when
parents have applied their ideas with their child (they may have been
able to come up with some very useful ideas to overcome difficult problems). Once you have reviewed all the positive aspects of parents' efforts
with their child, remind them that now it will be important for their
child to take the lead. You can introduce humor and your own difficulties when teaching this strategy as a way of demonstrating how difficult
it can be to keep good ideas to yourself and not take over. For example:
"It's so tricky to not share good ideas when working on a problem. I find
this happens all the time when I'm teaching the strategy, and sometimes
I literally have to bite my tongue! Do you find this difficult? Ultimately,
we want your child to become independent in his/her problem-solving
ability, so it's best to let the child have a go, no matter how strange some
of the ideas might be or how much you sometimes disagree with those
ideas."

TAKE-HOME MESSAGES

✓ Problem solving is a very useful strategy for realistic anxious thoughts or thoughts that reflect situations that may, in fact, happen.

✓ Problem solving helps children (and parents) develop a sense of being able to cope in different situations.

✓ Teaching parents how to problem-solve is a useful way of conveying the strategy so that they can then help their child to become an independent problem solver.

HANDOUT 7.1. Problem-Solving Worksheet

What is the problem?	What could I do?	What would happen if I did this?	Rating (0–10)	
			How good would this be?	How easy would this be to do?

CHAPTER 8

Keeping Things Going

Once all the key strategies have been shared with parents and they have had an opportunity to practice the tasks at home, parents may assume that the work has been completed. However, the formal parts of this treatment (i.e., the sessions with a therapist) are really only the beginning. Although it is common for some noticeable gains to have been made over the course of the program, given that this is a brief treatment, we do not expect all the goals to have been achieved by this point, or for the child to have recovered completely. If parents have understood the skills, feel confident about using them, and have a plan in place to work toward their goals, further gains can be achieved going forward without the need for ongoing therapist support. This independent application of the program requires continued commitment by the parents as well as considered and realistic planning. For these reasons, scheduling dedicated time with the therapist, during which parents develop plans for "keeping things going," is essential. Specifically, time needs to be spent encouraging parents by reflecting on the gains that have been made so far and what has made those achievements possible. Consideration of the goals to focus on next and how to achieve them is also critical.

What the Evidence Tells Us

Can Parents Expect to See Continued Improvement Over Time?

A review of studies that have assessed outcomes in children more than 2 years after they were treated for childhood anxiety disorders (2 years old to 7 years, 4 months, posttreatment) showed maintenance of or further improvement in children's outcomes after cognitive-behavioral approaches had been employed (Nevo & Manassis, 2009). With regard to guided parent-delivered CBT specifically, continued improvements have also been found 6 months (Thirlwall & Creswell, 2010) and up to 4 years after treatment was completed (Brown, Thirlwall, & Creswell, 2016). Although these studies could not determine whether the ongoing application of CBT strategies or other confounding influences, such as maturation, influenced the course of recovery, anxious symptoms were typically stable in untreated preadolescent children (Simon, van der Sluis, Muris, Thompson, & Cartwright-Hatton, 2014), suggesting that the further gains achieved beyond the end of treatment were at least partly due to ongoing use of the strategies learned in treatment. This notion is also supported by the finding that treatments where parents are shown how to implement CBT strategies at home (i.e., the transfer of control is passed from the therapist to the parent) and are taught specific skills in contingency management (i.e., ways to reinforce and encourage their child's positive behaviors) are more likely to be associated with long-term maintenance of treatment gains compared to those that do not include these elements (Manassis et al., 2014). Taken together, the literature suggests that parents can expect to see continued improvement in their child's anxiety after the end of treatment. However, the continual implementation of the strategies learned is likely to play a key role in this positive outcome.

What Are the Goals?

- To highlight the key strategies discussed in this book.
- To help parents reflect on what has been helpful for their family.
- To encourage parents to continue implementing strategies that have been helpful.
- To establish goals for parents to work toward with their child in the short and long term.
- To problem-solve with parents any difficulties that may prevent them for continuing the work.
- To increase parents' confidence by recognizing their achievements.

How to Do It

Overview of Strategies

It is important to provide a brief overview of the key strategies discussed during the previous sessions. The list below provides an outline of these and some of the key themes.

Providing Psychoeducation (Chapter 3)

Parents had opportunities to discuss factors that are potentially keeping their child's difficulties with anxiety going. The implications for treatment will have been discussed and parents will have been encouraged to think about which aspects of the treatment may be particularly pertinent to their child to best help the child overcome his or her difficulties.

Encouraging Independence and Promoting "Have a Go" Behavior (Chapter 4)

Parents will have been encouraged to consider the importance of increasing the child's independence in order to help the child gain confidence in trying things for him- or herself in nonemotive contexts and for the parents to experience supporting their child in succeeding at challenges. Strategies for parents to use to encourage their child to engage in "have a go" behavior, rather than avoiding his or her fears, will have been shared. These included noticing and praising their child's efforts, rewarding brave behavior, and modeling their own brave behavior.

Encouraging "Have a Go" Thinking (Chapter 5)

Next, parents were taught new ways of responding to their child's worries to help their child think more flexibly and consider alternative perspectives. Instead of providing reassurance, parents were coached in asking their child questions in order to identify what he or she is thinking and to open up the possibility that other outcomes might be possible. The idea is for parents to "sow the seeds of doubt" in the child regarding his or her fearful expectations as a way to encourage the child to engage in exposure activities.

Helping Children Face Their Fears (Chapter 6)

Parents learned a lot about how avoidance can maintain their child's anxiety, and they were supported in helping their child face his or her fear by taking a step-by-step approach toward their goal and discussing what had been learned from these experiences.

Helping Parents Promote Problem Solving (Chapter 7)

At times, children may face problems that need to be tackled, or they may be left with residual concerns that something bad *might* happen. At these times, it is important for children to be able to feel they can deal with difficulties independently (which might include seeking appropriate help, if needed). Parents will have practiced helping their child recognize when there is a problem and how to generate and evaluate solutions before ultimately putting them in to place.

Any other specific strategies—for example, for school refusal or sleep problems—should also be reviewed and discussed at this stage.

What Has Been Helpful?

It is vital to give parents an opportunity to reflect on what have been the most useful strategies thus far and what they will use going forward. There will be some skills that the child has found beneficial and some that he or she doesn't like or that simply don't "fit" with the family. If parents raise concern or doubts over any particular skill, make sure they have understood it correctly and implemented the techniques in line with your discussions; then make gentle suggestions as to how these strategies could be tweaked if applicable. Often parents identify other useful strategies during the course of treatment that may not have been a direct part of the treatment program. Give parents time to reflect on any other things that they have discovered that seem to work for them and their child. It is sometimes surprising what parents mention, and these discoveries need to be acknowledged and the parents' efforts celebrated.

> Useful Questions to Ask Parents
>
> ➤ "Which strategies have helped your child the most? Which ones have he or she responded well to?"
> ➤ "What do you think you have done well and how has this impacted on your child?"

Sticking Point

"The parents feel as though they haven't made much progress at all. They seem disheartened and unsure whether to continue."

If the child has made good progress and the parents have made good use of the strategies, we would not typically offer further treatment sessions but would encourage the parents to continue to put the strategies in place. Sometimes parents will raise concern about their child's residual problems and what will happen next. Often parents will expect that their child should have made a full recovery at the end of their sessions with a therapist, and this may not have happened. Be sure to emphasize that children will not always have made a full recovery within such a short treatment, but that often families need to have more time and opportunities to practice and implement the strategies in their daily life. Remind parents that they have had to take on board a lot of information and many strategies in a relatively short period of time, and that now you are at the end of treatment they have the opportunity to bring it all together and apply these strategies consistently to relevant situations. It is also possible that parents may have overlooked important advances that their child has made. It is important to review earlier notes and outcome measures and to compare these to how things are now. You can also remind parents of some of the achievements they have told you about in previous sessions.

Discussing Progress

The parent's level of motivation following treatment will be influenced by how much their child's anxiety problems have improved. For this reason it is essential that time is spent on both highlighting the progress that has already been made and encouraging parents to continue with the work, irrespective of whether they have achieved all the goals that were set or not.

Useful Questions to Ask Parents

➤ "Since you started this treatment, what progress has your child made in overcoming some of his or her fears and worries?"

➤ "Do you envisage any future challenges? What can you do to prevent these from causing any setbacks?"

Identifying Future Goals

To promote ongoing practice and further progress, parents should be asked to identify one or more goals to continue to work on with their child. Ideally, these will include both short- and long-term goals, with a clear plan for which will be tackled first. It is important to help parents begin to generate a clear plan for their first goal, including drafting a plan for graded exposure. Encourage the parents to write down these goals in the session and to leave blank spaces for them to take home and finalize with their child and other family members, if applicable. Encourage parents to put these goals somewhere visible and to regularly review whether or not the goals have been achieved. Ask parents if there might be any challenges to their doing this (e.g., having a busy schedule or forgetting) and help them to problem-solve these, using the steps outlined in Chapter 7, if necessary.

Celebrating Success

End the session by congratulating parents on their dedication and commitment over the course of the program. It is important to highlight the fact that you, the therapist, has not worked directly with the child, so it is clear that all the gains that have been made are a direct result of the work the parent has done.

Model praise and outline what the parent has done well, using specific examples (e.g., "I've been particularly impressed by how you have persisted with the exposure plan, despite Amy's being quite resistant to trying the steps. Because you kept going and tried hard to find motivating rewards, Amy did confront her fears!"). At this point we often encourage parents to take this opportunity to mark the success they have had and to reward themselves in a clear way. For example, some parents who had previously not been able to leave their child with a babysitter might go out for a meal; others have said they will just have a nice relaxing bath!

Time for Questions

As this is the last session, it is important to leave time for any questions that parents may raise and for them not to feel rushed. Often parents will want to know whether they can contact you if needed and what they should do if things deteriorate in the future. It is important to have thought through how you might respond to these questions beforehand, within the constraints posed by your service. Where possible, our preference is to be able to "keep the door open" for parents to make contact by phone or e-mail. If substantial difficulties emerge, the family may need to be "re-referred" to the service, but in many cases they just want to run their ideas for how to overcome a particular roadblock by us to prevent problems from escalating.

TAKE-HOME MESSAGES

✓ Parents are now equipped with strategies to help their child overcome their difficulties with anxiety.

✓ With practice and ongoing use of these strategies, it is likely that the child will make further progress.

✓ The family will be helped to stay on track by setting short- and long-term goals and reviewing them regularly.

✓ Parents should be encouraged to notice and celebrate the progress that has been made through their hard work.

CHAPTER 9

Tackling Sleep Problems

Sleep problems are very common in children with anxiety difficulties and come in several forms. Some children find it hard to get to sleep and lay awake for several hours before falling asleep. Other children are not able to settle to sleep by themselves and may want a parent's comfort in the night if they wake. Sometimes children are not able to sleep alone at all and either sleep in their parent's bed or in their parent's room. For most, although not all families, any form of sleep disruption is problematic and interferes significantly in the family's everyday life. These types of sleep difficulties are typically a behavioral response to heightened anxiety. For example, the child may be fearful of being alone and thus tries to avoid this circumstance by demanding the presence of his or her parent at bedtime or during the night. Other sleep difficulties often relate to generalized anxiety wherein falling asleep becomes difficult due to excessive worrying and increased arousal at bedtime. Other types of sleep problems include nightmares and night terrors.

Childhood sleep problems are incredibly disruptive to both the child and family. The child often does not get enough sleep, which results in further difficulties, such as excessive tiredness, poor concentration, or increased irritability. For parents, it may mean spending up to several hours each evening sitting with their child as he or she goes to sleep or being woken up repeatedly during the night.

Sleep difficulties may resolve as a result of addressing anxiety issues using the strategies already outlined in this book. However, in many cases, we suggest that tackling sleep problems should be a priority, given the high level of interference for the family, and that the child (and parent) may find other anxiety management strategies harder to implement if sleep-deprived.

Using CBT strategies to address sleep issues often results in less, rather than more, sleep initially and requires a very high level of commitment by parents, so it is important to ensure that they are committed to making changes and that you are explicit about the challenges that they may face. Parents are key to any successful sleep intervention; in our experience it is extremely difficult to tackle a sleep-related difficulty without parental input, and thus this parent-led program is well suited to overcoming this type of problem.

This chapter initially outlines the evidence that supports a CBT approach for sleep difficulties and the goals for this work, and then discuss assessment of sleep difficulties. We also address sleep hygiene and how to support parents in improving sleep hygiene for their child before tailoring the CBT strategies already discussed in this book to specifically tackle sleep problems.

What the Evidence Tells Us

Do All Anxious Children Have Problems with Sleeping?

Sleep problems are very common in anxious children, with 88% of youth experiencing at least one sleep-related problem (Alfano, Ginsburg, & Kingery, 2007). Sleep problems are also associated with impairments in daily functioning, confirming the high level of interference caused by such difficulties (Storch et al., 2008). Similarly, acute and cumulative loss of sleep results in increased levels of fear and anxiety the next day, indicating a vicious cycle that perpetuates the anxiety problem (Dinges et al., 1997; Leotta, Carskadon, Acebo, Seifer, & Quinn, 1997)—a further reason for making sleep problems the initial focus of treatment.

Is There an Association between the Type of Anxiety Problem a Child Experiences and Sleep Difficulties?

Studies have found that children with GAD and separation anxiety disorder have more sleep problems, as reported by their parents, than children with other types of anxiety problems, such as social anxiety disorder (Alfano, Pina, Zerr, & Villalta, 2010; Alfano & Mellman, 2010), with 87% of children with GAD and 60% with separation anxiety disorder reporting difficulties with sleep. Children with separation anxiety commonly find it hard to sleep without a parent/sibling present or close by due to their separation fears, whereas children with GAD often worry excessively at bedtime, which leads to delayed sleep latency.

How Do a Child's Anxiety Problems Result in Trouble Sleeping?

Cognitive arousal at bedtime is associated with greater sleep problems and less sleep overall (Alfano et al., 2010). In other words, a child who experiences excessive and uncontrollable worry at bedtime will find it harder to get to sleep and gain less sleep than a child who does not experience these types of difficulties. These findings were specific to cognitive but not somatic arousal, suggesting that the cognitive elements of anxiety are more likely to affect sleep patterns than the child's physiological state. In line with these findings, we do not routinely use relaxation as a strategy to manage sleep difficulties in anxious children.

Does CBT Work for Sleep Difficulties?

Behavioral treatments for sleep problems have typically included similar components to those used in CBT packages for use with anxious children: that is, techniques aimed at reducing anxious thinking and addressing avoidance and relaxation, supplemented with advice to improve sleep hygiene. There have been few studies investigating the efficacy of CBT for sleep problems specifically in the context of anxiety difficulties in children. One study used a 14-week CBT program and found a significant improvement in parent-reported child sleep difficulties (Storch et al., 2008). Two further studies used a brief CBT intervention and reported improvements in sleep and anxiety (Paine & Gradisar, 2011; Schlarb, Velten-Schurian, Poets, & Hautzinger, 2011). Finally, a study aimed at treating both GAD and sleep problems reported positive outcomes for both sleep and anxiety in a published case series (Clementi & Alfano, 2014). This intervention involved both individual child sessions and sessions with the parent and child. The authors highlighted the importance of parents in establishing healthy sleep habits and helping children to develop nighttime self-regulatory strategies.

What Are the Goals?

- To ensure that parents have a good understanding of their child's sleep problem.
- To provide an opportunity for parents to evaluate their child's sleep hygiene and to make changes if problem areas are identified.
- To support parents in adapting and implementing CBT strategies (outlined in previous chapters) so that they can be used effectively to tackle the child's sleep problems.

How to Do It

Assessing Sleep Problems

Your structured anxiety assessment will have provided some information about the child's sleep patterns. However, we would recommend that you ask additional questions about the child's sleep difficulties to ensure that you have a comprehensive understanding.

Useful Questions to Ask Parents

➤ "What time does your child go to bed?"

➤ "What time does your child fall asleep?"

➤ "Does your child worry excessively at bedtime?"

➤ "What does your child do when he or she worries (e.g., calls out, goes to the toilet repeatedly, reads a book)?"

➤ "Can your child fall asleep alone, or does he or she need a parent/ other present?"

➤ "Does your child awaken in the night? If so, when and how often?"

➤ "What does your child do when he or she awakens?"

➤ "What do you/others do if your child wakes?"

➤ "Does your child worry about the effect of not sleeping on what he or she is doing the next day?"

➤ "Does your child worry about not sleeping the following night?"

In addition, there are a number of standardized questionnaires that assess sleep difficulties in children, including the Children's Sleep Habits Questionnaire (CSHQ; Owens, Spirito, & McGuinn, 2001) and the Sleep Disturbance Scale for Children (SDSC; Bruni et al., 1997). Both are relatively short parent-report questionnaires that include 45 and 27 items, respectively, to assess a range of sleep difficulties, including bedtime behavior and sleep onset, sleep duration, anxiety around sleep, nightmares, and sleep-disordered breathing. The Sleep Self Report (SSR; Owens, Spirito, McGuinn, & Nobile, 2000), a 26-item questionnaire designed as a self-report measure for children 7–12 years of age, measures similar domains to the CSHQ.

A sleep diary is also helpful to gather more detailed information about the child's sleep pattern on a daily basis. We recommend that you tailor the diary to the type of difficulties the particular child presents with, using the information you have just collected by asking the questions suggested above in order to do so.

Case Examples

Seven-year-old Lily is an only child who lives with both parents. Her parents report that, for as long as they can remember, she has always been clingy toward her mother and has needed her mother to sit with her until she falls asleep. Sometimes Lily wakes in the night and comes into her parents' bed, where she sleeps for the rest of the night. Lily does not like going upstairs alone and never plays in her bedroom by herself. She has told her mother that she is worried there will be an intruder in the house who will hurt her and her family.

Eleven-year-old Tom has GAD. He lives with his mother and two older brothers and sees his father every other weekend. Tom worries about lots of things at bedtime, but particularly that he won't be able to sleep and will be too tired the next day. Tom lies awake in bed for up to 2 or 3 hours at night and is always tired in the morning. He has tried lots of different ways to help himself sleep (e.g., reading/audiobooks, going to bed earlier), but none has worked. Tom worries that he will get reprimanded at school if he is tired as he may fall asleep. He also worries he won't do well with his work and may have a bad game when he is playing football.

Could the Child's Sleep Hygiene Be Improved?

Sleep hygiene refers to aspects of a lifestyle and bedtime routine that could be changed to improve the individual's sleep pattern (Espie, 2006). We recommend that the first step to tackling sleep difficulties is to assess and monitor the child's sleep and bedtime-related habits, as some of the factors highlighted in the following sections may be maintaining or exacerbating the child's sleep difficulties.

Lifestyle

Diet and exercise can influence how a child sleeps. Both hunger and being overly full can cause wakefulness and make it harder to get to sleep. Parents should be asked to consider whether their child might be hungry at bedtime, and if so, introduce a small snack at that time. If the child may be overly full, they will need to restrict the amount of food that is eaten immediately before bed or move dinner to an earlier time. Caffeine is also well known to cause wakefulness, so it is important to check that the child is not drinking large quantities of caffeine-filled drinks during the day or any caffeine close to bedtime.

There is good evidence of a link between exercise, fitness, and sleep quality, so it is important to discuss with the parent how much exercise the child gets. If the child is not particularly athletic and thus does not naturally engage in regular exercise, it is worth talking to the parent about identifying a physical activity that the child would be happy to engage in and how to schedule this in each day (although not too late in the day, as strenuous exercise close to bedtime can lead to difficulties getting to sleep).

Bedtime Routine

Loud and/or sudden noises can affect a child's ability to get to and stay asleep. We recommend that you explore with the parent ways to keep noise levels to a minimum at night time. Room temperature can also affect sleep. Check out with the parent if the child might be too hot or too cold and discuss how to resolve this if it is a problem. Similarly, check out if the child's bed is comfortable or if he or she is complaining of being uncomfortable in bed.

Lighting can be a significant issue for anxious children. In our experience, many children in this age group who have significant anxiety at bedtime use a night-light or ask for a nearby light to be left on. Although this often helps to reduce a child's anxiety, light can have a significant affect on a child's ability to go to sleep. If the child does have a night-light or other light on at night, discuss with the parent whether this may be affecting the child's ability to get to sleep, and try to find an alternative solution—for example, using a smaller or dimmer light, working toward not having a light on at all.

There is good evidence that having time to "wind down" before going to bed can be beneficial for good quality sleep. We suggest that the parent starts this winding-down process approximately an hour before the child is due to go to bed. There has been much debate in recent years about the contributory role of computers and handheld screens in delaying sleep. We thus recommend that the hour wind-down time does not involve any computer or screen-related activities. Discuss with the parent what the child can do to wind down and relax and how the parent can support this process. Ideas might include listening to a story, listening to music, taking a bath, reading a book, doing some coloring, or engaging in other calming activities.

Although these strategies may not resolve a sleep problem alone, they will ensure that you have addressed factors that may be contributing to the sleep issue, prior to embarking on a CBT intervention with the parent.

Sticking Point

"I am not sure the parents are really motivated to tackle their child's sleep problem? What can I do?"

Typically, parents are highly motivated to overcome a child's sleep problem. However, there are times when a child's inability to sleep independently brings some benefits to parents, for example, if they do not have a partner, and enjoy the physical comfort of their child close by, or perhaps if marital relations are strained, and a child's sleep problems thus allow both parents to avoid facing this issue. For other parents, they may have simply followed a particular course as it offers the least line of resistance, within the context of leading busy and often stressful lives.

It is thus important to fully understand parents' goals for treatment and not to assume they want to tackle a sleep issue. However, encouraging a child to sleep independently is an appropriate developmental goal in many cultures and will only serve to increase the child's sense of confidence in their ability to cope, and we would thus recommend that you consider this with parents. Some parents may feel guilty or to blame for their child's sleep difficulties so, as always, it is critical that the therapist recognizes that many parental responses that may inadvertently maintain sleep difficulties are perfectly normal and understandable reactions that may be effective with some children in some circumstances (e.g., sitting with a child while they go to sleep).

Applying CBT Techniques to Sleep Problems

Promoting Independence and "Have a Go" Behavior

All the strategies outlined in Chapter 4 are applicable to children with sleep problems, particularly the use of praise and rewards. A child with a sleep problem may not necessarily be motivated to overcome this difficulty and may be likely to prefer the idea of staying with his or her parent at night. As such, the use of praise and rewards is crucial to increase the child's motivation to overcome his or her fear.

If sleeping independently and away from the parent is the agreed-upon goal, then developing independence in other areas is also a good idea because it will only serve to increase the child's confidence and promote beliefs that he or she can cope without additional help (see Chapter 4).

It might be helpful to encourage children with GAD who have sleep-related worries to follow the "Worry Box" strategies, and to talk to their parent about these worries at an agreed-upon time—"Worry Time" (see Chapter 4)—to promote independence in dealing with their worries and a sense of control over them. However, it is important that the child's worries are not discussed close to bedtime because it may interfere with his or her ability to settle to sleep.

Encouraging "Have a Go" Thinking

As outlined in Chapter 5, parents need to establish a good understanding of their child's negative expectations toward sleep or bedtime. These may include thoughts that someone will come into the child's home and hurt either the child or the parent or both of them. Sometimes younger children worry that there may be a monster in the house that will scare and/or hurt them. The role of the parent is then to support the child in seeing these thoughts as possibilities (rather than facts) and to encourage curiosity about them (using the techniques described in Chapter 5) so that the child develops openness to testing out the fears. Parents often ask about the timing of such an exercise. We suggest that the parent does this earlier in the evening or after school, because engaging in a discussion about the child's worries at bedtime may be counterproductive to the goal of settling the child to sleep more quickly.

As we describe in Chapter 5 (sticking points), some children will not have any information or experiences to draw on to help them consider that there might be other possibilities aside from their negative expectations. In these circumstances, the parent may need to help the child gather more information that would ultimately help him or her feel able to put the fear to the test. For example, a child might design a survey for family or friends to report on whether they have experienced a burglary and, if so, how they coped. Alternatively, a child could search the house to find out what is causing the strange noise that he or she often hears at nighttime.

Figure 9.1 is an example of a handout that Lily's mother completed after she had tried to encourage "have a go" thinking with Lily.

Exposure Tasks

We highly recommend using exposure to address sleep problems related to separation anxiety. In fact, this is probably the most important aspect of a CBT intervention for this type of sleep problem (see Chapter 6). In doing so, children are likely to gradually change their expectations about

What is happening?	What is the child thinking? (e.g., Why are you worried?; What do you think will happen?; What is it about [this situation] that is making you worried?)	Acknowledge the child's struggle/Label his or her emotion (e.g., Yes, that would make anyone feel nervous; That must be difficult; Most people would be upset by x too if they thought that; Gosh, that does sound like a frightening thought.)	Ask questions (e.g., What makes you think that [this situation] will happen?; Has that happened to you before?; Have you seen that happen to someone else?; What has happened before [to you/other people])?; What would [someone else] think would happen if he or she was in this situation?)	Promote curiosity (e.g., That's interesting, isn't it?; So, I wonder what would actually happen?; So, it is possible it may happen like that or may not—it's hard to know, I suppose.)
Lily doesn't want to go to sleep by herself.	I asked Lily what she thought might happen—she said, "Maybe there is someone there." I asked who, and she said, "Maybe a strange man or a nasty person."	I said, "That would be scary, wouldn't it?" Lily said, "That's why I want to stay with you," and I said, "I can understand that."	I asked, "What makes you think there will be a nasty man in the house?" Lily said, "I just think there will be. You hear things on the news about nasty people, don't you?" I asked. "Has it happened to you before? Have you seen someone?" Lily said, "No, never, but I think it might." I asked, "Has it happened to your friends or any of your family? Have they seen someone in their house?" Lily said, "No, I don't think so."	I reflected with Lily that it was impossible to be sure what will happen at nighttime and Lily agreed.

FIGURE 9.1. "Have a go" thinking with Lily.

the feared situation and learn that they can cope without their parent close by at nighttime.

The ultimate goal is almost always for the child to sleep independently. However, this is sometimes too difficult an exposure task for the child initially, because it will lead to very high levels of anxiety and to the child becoming highly distressed and inevitably refusing to even attempt it again. A graded exposure plan can be devised to enable the child to engage in exposure tasks in a manageable way (see Figure 9.2 for an example of a sleep exposure plan for Lily). This graded exposure can be set up in a number of ways for children who are dependent on their parent being with them until they are able to sleep on their own throughout the night. The plan can involve either a gradual physical separation from the child (i.e., the parent gradually moves further away from the child's room until he or she is engaging in normal evening activities) or a gradual reduction of time in the bedroom with the child (i.e., the parent initially checks on the child frequently, and then the frequency of the checking is gradually reduced). If the parent and child are sleeping in the same room all night, the former exposure plan is more practical, although it may involve sleeping on a mattress in the hall or close to the child's room for a period of time. It is usually better to have the parent move gradually out of the child's room rather than moving the child out of the parent's room so that the child is getting used to being in his or her own room from the start. As described in Chapter 6, it is important to encourage the parent to ask the child for his or her prediction before completing a step, and then to reflect on what actually happened, how the child coped, and what he or she learned from the experience.

The parent can also encourage the child to use one or more coping strategies at bedtime (e.g., listening to an audiobook) and gradually removing these could also form part of the step plan. The parent can use problem solving (see "Problem Solving" on page 155 and Chapter 7) to support the child in generating his or her own coping strategies at this time.

Exposure tasks can also be used for children with sleep-related GAD worries to test out their negative expectations that they may not be able to cope with whatever they fear. For example, a child with GAD may be worried that he or she cannot cope without their mother's support at bedtime because the worries are too upsetting, so the child calls for their mother multiple times each night. A series of graded exposure tasks might include the child's calling for their mother fewer and fewer times, until the child reaches the ultimate goal of not calling for their mother at all and managing his or her worries independently at bedtime. Problem solving (see "Problem Solving" on page 155 and Chapter 7) can be used to help children develop strategies to manage their bedtime worries without help from their parents.

Ultimate Goal	To settle to sleep alone with Mom and Dad downstairs	
Reward	Family trip to the movies to celebrate my success!	
Step 8	For Mom and Dad to come and check on me once only after a ½ hour	
Reward	Bedtime 15 minutes later	
Step 7	For Mom and Dad to go to the living room but to come and check on me every 20 minutes	
Reward	10 minutes on my computer game in the morning	
Step 6	For Mom and Dad to go to the living room but to come and check on me every 10 minutes	
Reward	New poster for my bedroom	
Step 5	For Mom and Dad to go to the living room but to come and check on me every 7 minutes	
Reward	Bedtime 10 minutes later	
Step 4	For Mom and Dad to go to the living room but to come and check on me every 5 minutes	
Reward	A new bedroom lamp	
Step 3	To settle to sleep with Mom or Dad sitting on the bottom of the stairs	
Reward	Bedtime 5 minutes later	
Step 2	To settle to sleep with Mom or Dad sitting on the landing	
Reward	Favorite breakfast cereal	
Step 1	To settle to sleep with Mom or Dad sitting by my door	
Reward	Praise from Mom and Dad	

FIGURE 9.2. Exposure plan for Lily: Sleep problems.

Exposure tasks can also be carried out individually, alongside a graded exposure plan. For example, a child with GAD who is worried about performing badly at school the next day because of not getting to sleep early enough, accepts an invitation to go to the cinema with a friend in the evening or stays up late with his dad to watch a football match on TV. Similarly, a child with separation anxiety could go for a sleepover with her grandparents.

Problem Solving

Problem solving is a useful strategy to help children find ways to manage their sleep-related difficulties or to help them feel able to cope with feared situations that might possibly occur. Chapter 7 gives a detailed account of the strategy. For example, parents can problem-solve with their child to consider different strategies to use when the child is lying in bed and finding it hard to control his or her worries, or they can problem-solve what the child could do if an intruder came into the house (even if it is unlikely). This approach often gives children a sense of control over the situation and helps them consider the possibility that they could cope even if the worst-case scenario occurred. Figure 9.3 is an example of Tom's problem-solving worksheet. Having completed the problem solving, he decided to try out the solution "Write down my worries to talk about with Mom and Dad the next day."

Parents can also use problem solving themselves to overcome a whole host of problems that they might face as result of their child's sleep problem (e.g., "How do we cope with lack of sleep while we are tackling this issue?"; "How do I ensure that I'll wake up when my child gets into bed with me in the middle of the night?").

Figure 9.4 is an example of a problem that Lily's parents decided to tackle using problem solving. Having completed this process, they decided that there were two equally good solutions and so agreed to implement both, taking it in turns to do each step and asking Lily's grandmother to have the children on a Saturday so they could get some rest.

Other Considerations

Nightmares and night terrors are often classified alongside sleep walking as "parasomnias," and some studies (e.g., Alfano et al., 2010) have found higher rates of these types of behaviors in children with separation anxiety and GAD, whereas other studies (e.g., Reynolds & Alfano, 2016) have not.

What is the problem?	What could I do?	What would happen if I did this?	Rating (0–10)	
			How good would this be?	How easy would this be to do?
When I'm in bed, my worries are really bad and stop me from sleeping.	Read a book.	I have tried this a lot and I can't concentrate on the books, as my worries take over.	3	7
	Call Mom or Dad.	They would help me feel better, but once they leave, I will start worrying again.	5	10
	Listen to some music.	It would probably help, although I will probably still worry a bit.	6	8
	Write down my worries to talk about with Mom or Dad the next day.	It would take my mind off my worries, as I would know I will get to talk about them.	8	7

FIGURE 9.3. Tom's Problem-Solving Worksheet.

What is the problem?	What could I do?	What would happen if I did this?	Rating (0–10)	
			How good would this be?	How easy would this be to do?
We won't be able to cope with getting even less sleep while we work on Lily's sleep problems.	We could take it in turns to do each step so one of us gets some sleep every other night.	We would get some sleep. It might work better to both do the plan anyway, but we would still be a bit sleep deprived.	8	9
	We could take some time off work and sleep in the day.	We would have used up quite a bit of our leave and may not be able to sleep in the day, but we would be less tired.	5	5
	We could just put up with the lack of sleep, as it won't last forever.	We could probably do this for a week but might struggle if it went on for longer, and we might end up giving up on the plan in order to get some sleep.	4	3
	We could ask my mom to take the kids on Saturday so we can have a rest and maybe get some sleep.	Mom would agree to this and at least we could have a quiet day and maybe have a short nap, which would help for facing the next few nights.	7	10

FIGURE 9.4. Lily's parents' Problem-Solving Worksheet.

Parent-led CBT for anxiety difficulties may well have a positive impact on these types of sleep problems, in the context of child anxiety, because they are likely to reduce as a child's overall anxiety level decreases.

TAKE-HOME MESSAGES

✓ Sleep problems are very common in anxious children.

✓ Children tend to experience one of two types of sleep issues: worrying excessively at nighttime or having difficulties sleeping independently.

✓ Ensure that the child has good sleep hygiene before using CBT techniques.

✓ CBT strategies for anxiety can be adapted to work effectively for this type of problem.

CHAPTER 10

Tackling School Refusal

Given that the most common response to an anxiety-provoking situation is avoidance, it is not surprising that some children are so fearful of school or school-related situations that they begin to refuse to attend, and some become "school refusers." School refusal behavior is defined as "child-motivated refusal to attend school or difficulties remaining in school for an entire day" (Kearney & Silverman, 1996, p. 345). It creates enormous difficulties both for the child and parent. There is a significant impact from not accessing education, seeing friends, or engaging in other extracurricular activities, and also from the practical difficulty of having a child at home full time, the parental stress caused by having to deal with school authorities, and the potential legal consequences for parents.

The school environment presents a range of potentially anxiety-provoking situations for children. Attending school requires children to leave their parents and to encounter a very social environment that often places demands on children to interact with and speak or perform in front of peers. Thus it is understandable that children with separation and social anxiety often find that attending school is very difficult for them. Similarly, children with generalized anxiety often worry excessively about a range of school-related issues, including not being good enough at their work or at sports, mismanaging friendships, getting in trouble, or seemingly small everyday matters. Children with specific phobias can also find school highly anxiety-provoking; for example, those with a specific phobia of being exposed to the possibility of witnessing another child being sick or of catching unwanted germs.

Intervention studies have typically defined school refusal as being present when the child (1) displays persistent difficulties in attending school; (2) experiences severe emotional upset associated with attending school; (3) is at home with full knowledge of the parent when he or she should be at school; (4) shows no signs of antisocial characteristics (Berg, Nichols, & Pritchard, 1969). Few studies have evaluated treatments for anxiety-based school refusal, but CBT is the most well-evaluated treatment for this type of difficulty, with packages typically focussing on the types of strategies that we have described in this book. This chapter describes how these strategies can be applied effectively for anxiety-based school refusal and addresses a number of questions that parents commonly raise, including the potential advantages and disadvantages of changing schools and home tutoring.

What the Evidence Tells Us

Is School Refusal Common?

School refusal occurs in about 1% of all school-age children and in 5% of clinic-referred children (King, Ollendick, & Tonge, 1995). Rates are similar among boys and girls. The incidence of school refusal peaks at 5–6 years of age and again at 10–11 years, reflecting the ages that children typically commence primary and secondary grades (Ollendick & Mayer, 1984). School refusal is commonly associated with high levels of anxiety; for example, in one study, 22% of children exhibiting school refusal behavior met the criteria for separation anxiety disorder, and 10% met criteria for GAD (Kearney & Albano, 2004); in another study, around 50% of children met the criteria for an anxiety disorder (Walter et al., 2010). However, school refusal can also be associated with other emotional or behavioral difficulties, including oppositional behavior (8%) and low mood (5%) (Kearney & Albano, 2004), highlighting the importance of a robust assessment (see Chapter 2).

What Causes Some Children with Anxiety Difficulties to Refuse to Attend School, Whereas Others Are Able to Continue to Go to School Despite High Levels of Anxiety?

A number of factors may differentiate those children with anxiety difficulties who refuse to attend school from those who do attend school, despite their anxieties. Stressful life events, including the death of a parent or close relative or a change of school, have been found to commonly precede the onset of school refusal (Blagg, 1987; Hersov, 1960). Risk factors for the development of school absenteeism more generally have been identified and include the presence of an anxiety disorder, behavioral difficulties, substance abuse problems, higher psychiatric severity, and having a low number of close friends (Ingul & Nordahl, 2013).

Does CBT Work for Children with School Attendance Problems?

Unfortunately, there have only been a very small number of randomized controlled trials examining the efficacy of treatments for anxiety-related school refusal, but the outcomes are generally positive. King et al. (1998) delivered individual CBT to children ages 5–15 years with anxiety disorders and school refusal and found clinically significant improvements in school attendance compared to a wait-list control. However, a study comparing CBT to educational support found no significant differences in school attendance (Last, Hansen, & Franco, 1998). Of interest, younger children and those with a higher level of school refusal at baseline showed the greatest improvement, highlighting the importance of addressing school refusal early. A small number of other studies have examined the efficacy of interventions that included some cognitive and/or behavioral aspects (e.g., Blagg & Yule, 1984; Kearney & Silverman, 1996) and have provided some support for their use. Overall, it has been concluded that the small number of studies of psychosocial interventions have demonstrated positive and significant effects on school attendance, but have not significantly altered the child's anxiety symptoms in the short term (although this may have been a result of children's continuing anxious feelings while they continued to face their fears) (Maynard et al., 2015).

Is Parent-Led CBT Effective in Tackling School Refusal Difficulties?

Two studies have reported positive outcomes from CBT-based interventions for school refusal, in which parents were involved in either part or all of the intervention (King et al., 1998; Heyne et al., 2002). Both studies reported improvements in school attendance and reduced levels of anxiety following treatments that included parents. Of note, Heyne et al. compared child treatment to parent–teacher input and a combination of both interventions and found that children whose parents had been involved in treatment (with or without child-focused interventions) attended school more often than those who had not had parent involvement in the treatment. However, by the follow-up assessment there were no significant differences between the three groups. The authors concluded that working with parents alone, or children alone, may be sufficient to treat school refusal, and that a combined approach is not necessarily needed but that including parents may achieve good outcomes more quickly. They noted that working with parents may be particularly advantageous for younger children or for those who exhibit comorbid oppositional behavior, and when child anxiety symptoms are less severe.

What Are the Goals?

- To guide the parents in fully understanding what is maintaining their child's anxiety about attending school.
- To support the parents in applying a range of CBT strategies to their child's anxieties about school attendance.
- To support the parents in liaising effectively with the school (and other agencies) to ensure a team approach to the child's attendance difficulties.

How to Do It

How to Apply CBT Techniques to School Refusal

Promoting Independence and "Have a Go" Behavior

Not attending school can lead to a general reduction in children's independence. For example, they will not need to organize themselves and or necessarily complete daily routines in the morning, they may not need to complete homework, and they may lose the opportunity to walk to school independently. The guidance in Chapter 4 can be used to support parents in promoting their children's everyday independence skills, particularly those skills and activities that are needed for children to function well in school. This focus can help ensure that children are well prepared for their return to school as well as addressing concerns that they will not be able to cope without their parent being with them.

CASE EXAMPLE

Ten-year-old Laura lives with her parents and her younger sister, Eloise. Laura experiences social anxiety; she is shy and finds it hard to talk to her friends, so sometimes she feels left out. She is quiet in class and does not put her hand up or ask for help, hates doing presentations and speaking in front of her class, and also finds it really hard to say anything out loud in assembly. It's no surprise that Laura finds it hard to go to parties and after-school clubs and prefers to spend her time at home. She has always struggled with anxiety around attending school, but she has recently become more anxious in response to a substitute teacher who has been quite strict. Laura has now refused to go to school for several weeks, despite her mother's efforts to get her to go each day. Laura did manage to go for 1 day, but her friends asked her lots of questions about why she was not in school for so long, and one of the boys called her a "slacker," which has made her more worried about going back.

Praise and rewards are an important part of any CBT intervention for school refusal, and, in our experience, the use of a structured reward system for school attendance can work really well. However, the goals need to feel attainable to the child, and thus rewarding the child for attending school for a full week following a period of sustained absenteeism is likely to fail. We discuss graded exposure and how to use this technique successfully to address school attendance issues in "Exposure Tasks" on page 164.

Modeling brave behavior and confidence is also an important component of working with parents on school refusal issues because it is crucial that parents are able to model confident behavior in their interactions with school personnel. These opportunities may arise by attending school meetings or talking to a teacher on the telephone, or perhaps talking to the child's friends or the friends' parents. Similarly, it is crucial that parents are able to balance acknowledging the child's feelings with giving positive messages about attending school, both in terms of the importance, value, and potential fun in attending school and in terms of the parents' perceptions of the child's ability to cope with the challenges it will bring.

The following excerpt illustrates Laura's mother talking to her daughter in a way that promotes independence and models confidence:

"Laura, I spoke to your teacher today. She was really understanding about how hard things are for you. We talked about how important it is for you to get back to school; they are doing a project on World War II at the moment and Mrs. Smith thinks you will really enjoy it. We both said we were concerned that you don't miss too much work. Mrs, Smith also told me that your friends miss you. I know you feel worried about it, but I really think you can do it. You have Mrs. Smith and your friends on your side. You are a really determined person, and I know you can do something when you put your mind to it."

Encouraging "Have a Go" Thinking

As described in Chapter 5, the first step toward "have a go thinking" is to help parents identify their child's negative expectations. Although school refusal can be associated with a range of different negative expectations, persistent school nonattendance can lead to additional anxious thoughts, such as not being able to catch up with work, concern about being teased or repeatedly questioned by peers about the child's absence, and being seen as a truant or someone who "slacks off." As described in Chapter 5, helping parents promote "have a go" thinking is likely to be beneficial in encouraging the child to face his or her fears.

Sometimes children will not have enough information or experience to draw on to help them consider that there might be other possibilities aside from their negative expectations (see Chapter 5, Sticking Points on page 88). In these circumstances, parents may need to help their child gather more information that would ultimately help the child feel able to put the fears to the test. For example, a child who is worried that answering a question incorrectly in class would elicit laughter could do a survey at school for a week to see how many children get the answer wrong and how their peers react.

Figure 10.1 is an example of the handout that Laura's mother completed as part of encouraging her daughter to engage in "have a go" thinking.

Through discussing the child's negative expectations about returning to school or about particular school activities, it is possible that parents will become aware of specific challenges that the child has faced, or is facing, at school. For example, fears and worries about school may be associated with actual experiences of bullying, other challenging peer interactions, or difficulties with aspects of the work. In these cases, parents should take action, but they can still promote their child's autonomy by planning together, using a problem-solving approach (see "Problem Solving" on page 168 and Chapter 7), what and how this action should be accomplished.

Exposure Tasks

Graded exposure is a key part of any school refusal intervention. In fact, Heyne et al. (2002) concluded that it was the only common component across all three treatment conditions in his study, all of which produced excellent results. In the context of school refusal, exposure tasks tend to focus on reducing the child's avoidance of attending school and encouraging positive beliefs about coping with the challenges at school, in addition to encouraging the child to develop new learning in relation to his or her

What is happening?	What is the child thinking?	Acknowledge the child's struggle/Label his or her emotion	Ask questions	Promote curiosity
	(e.g., Why are you worried?; What do you think will happen?; What is it about [this situation] that is making you worried?)	(e.g., Yes, that would make anyone feel nervous; That must be difficult; Most people would be upset by x too if they thought that; Gosh, that does sound like a frightening thought.)	(e.g., What makes you think that [this situation] will happen?; Has that happened to you before?; Have you seen that happen to someone else?; What has happened before [to you/other people])?; What would [someone else] think would happen if he or she was in this situation?)	(e.g., That's interesting, isn't it?; So, I wonder what would actually happen?; So, it is possible it may happen like that or may not—it's hard to know, I suppose.)
Laura is worried what the other children will say when she goes back to school.	I asked, "What are you worried about?" Laura said, "I am not sure." I asked, "What do you think might happen?" and Laura said, "I think they will bug me, keep asking me questions."	I said, "That can be quite hard, can't it, if you do get asked a lot of questions?"	I asked, "What makes you think it will happen?" and Laura said, "When I went back for the day, Holly asked me lots of questions." I asked, "Did anything else happen when you went back for the day?", and Laura said, "Joe asked me a question too." I asked, "Did anyone else?", and Laura said, "No, they didn't. I asked, "What has happened to other children when they have been off and then come back?" and Laura said, "When Gail was away for a month, she got asked maybe one question—"Why were you off?"—I can't really remember now."	So I said to Laura, "It sounds like you and your friends do sometimes get asked questions when you have been out, but sometimes it is only one or two, although it's hard to know for certain, isn't it?

FIGURE 10.1. Example of the handout Laura's mother completed as part of encouraging her daughter to "have a go" thinking.

negative expectations. The principles of developing a graded exposure hierarchy are outlined in Chapter 6; here we describe how to apply these specifically to school refusal behavior. The goal for most school-refusal-related
hierarchies is full-time or part-time school attendance. Although the child
may not want this as a goal, both the parent and school personnel are very
likely to see attendance as a priority, so working directly with the parent can
be particularly advantageous in these circumstances.

The planned steps toward this goal will be different for each child. In
order to ascertain what these steps might be, parents need to find out from
the child how anxiety-provoking each aspect of school is for him or her. For
one child, break time or lunchtime may be most anxiety-provoking, due
to the unstructured and social nature of the environment, and thus this
may be a step that is placed near the top of the exposure plan. For another,
attending a lesson with a particular teacher might be the most difficult. For
other children, all aspects of the school day may be very anxiety-provoking,
and thus easier steps are required lower down the hierarchy, such as the
child putting on the school uniform but not actually attending school, driving or walking to school but not entering the school building, or staying in
the school office for the day. For children with separation anxiety, it may
not be a particular aspect of school that is anxiety-provoking, but rather
the fact that they will be away from their parents. In this case, a plan may
include a series of steps involving spending more time at school, and, if necessary, starting with time at school with a parent, and building up to time
at school without the parent present. For some children, having a parent
check in at certain times of day, or a planned phone call, can be helpful as
part of a systematic exposure plan.

As noted in Chapter 6, it is important for parents to encourage the
child to make predictions about what might happen when he or she carries
out each step and to review these predictions once the child has managed
to put them to the test.

School Liaison

Exposure plans related to school attendance can be difficult to put into
place because they usually require considerable coordination between the
family and school. Working directly with parents is very helpful in this
regard, because they are best placed to gain agreement on a plan with both
the child and the school. It is important that you encourage parents to
talk to key staff at their child's school as early as possible to begin to work
together to put a systematic plan of action into place. Ideally, we would

Sticking Point

"The parents are convinced that the child will not be motivated to work toward a goal of getting back to school. How can I help them to motivate the child?"

Support parents in how to talk with their child about why this is the planned goal. Parents should emphasize the paced approach of the plan to the child; that is, that it may take a while to achieve the ultimate goal and that they will progress at a pace that the child is able to manage. For example:

> "We believe that going to school is really important, not only for learning but also to see your friends, doing other things you enjoy (music, sports, etc.), and being independent from us. It is also the law that you go to school, so ultimately we have no choice but to support you in getting back into school. We know it is really hard for you at the moment, and we are not expecting you to go straight back. That is why we are working with x to help you feel less anxious and to work on your getting into school very gradually. So, although we have set your goal as getting into school full time, we know that will take a while, and you will have to build up to this slowly by doing school-related activities little by little. We really need your help to make this plan because only you know what scares you the most and the least about school."

Encourage the parents to explore with the child the pros and cons of attending school. For example, parents could ask the child to write down all the reasons why he or she doesn't want to go to school and all the reasons to go to school, thinking about both the short-term and the longer-term future.

Discuss with the parents the use of an interim goal that the child may find more manageable (e.g., attending favorite classes at school).

Use clearly defined rewards to increase the child's motivation to engage in this process.

encourage parents to meet with their child's teacher and possibly with the person in the school who oversees special needs that children may have (e.g., in the United Kingdom, most schools have a special educational needs coordinator [SENCO]), in order to fully discuss what a plan might look like and how, together, the parent and school might put this plan into place. Although the child's input will be crucial in terms of developing the plan, the motivation to put this into place is much more likely to come from both parents and school personnel.

Figure 10.2 is an example of Laura's exposure plan.

Alongside a graded exposure plan, parents can support the child in setting up individual exposure tasks to test out specific negative expectations related to school attendance (see Chapter 6). For a child who is fearful that he or she will get anxious when in a hot and busy classroom, an exposure task could be set up whereby the child spends half an hour in one of the hot classrooms in order to see how he or she copes. As noted, many children who refuse to attend school experience social anxiety. A number of common fears or negative expectations related to social anxiety include "Everyone will laugh at me if I read aloud in class" and "People will think I'm stupid if I put my hand up and get the wrong answer." Specific exposure tasks can be designed for each of these fears; for example, the child raises his or his hand and answers a question in an agreed-upon lesson and observes what happens or the child agrees to read out loud in class and observes how peers respond. However, the child will need to be able to attend school at least some of the time in order to carry out most of these tasks, so the tasks often work best alongside a graded exposure plan for attending school. Once again, it is important to gain the support of teaching staff in implementing a plan.

Problem Solving

Problem solving (see Chapter 7) can be a particularly useful tool for helping children plan how they will address difficulties in the school setting, where they often feel powerless to resolve the everyday problems that arise and where parents are not available for support. Problems can also arise as a result of their school nonattendance, as described in Laura's scenario above, that need to be resolved in order for a child to feel able to attend school.

Figure 10.3 is an example of a problem-solving handout completed by Laura with the help of her mother. Laura decided that the best solution would be to give Holly a brief answer and then talk about something else. She tried it out and her mom asked her how it went. Laura said that

Ultimate Goal	Attend school every day for a week	
Reward	Day out with a friend	
Step 9	Attend school every day but sit out of PE	
Reward	Get take-out food with friend	
Step 8	Attend all lessons but sit in library at lunchtime	
Reward	Half-day model-making session with Dad	
Step 7	Attend all classes but sit in library at break and lunchtime	
Reward	Have friend over for a sleepover	
Step 6	Attend all classes except for Mr. Daniel's PHSE lesson (and sit in library at break and lunch)	
Reward	Have friend over and rent a movie	
Step 5	Attend all classes up to lunchtime	
Reward	Go swimming with Mom	
Step 4	Attend first class every day	
Reward	Make favorite cake with Mom	
Step 3	Attend first class on Wednesday and Friday	
Reward	Buy a magazine	
Step 2	Attend first class on a Friday only	
Reward	Have a friend over to play after school	
Step 1	Come to school and meet Mrs. Smith	
Reward	Praise from Mom and Dad and have my favorite meal afterward	

FIGURE 10.2. Exposure plan for Laura: School refusal.

What is the problem?	What could I do?	What would happen if I did this?	Rating (0–10)	
			How good would this be?	How easy would this be to do?
Holly is going to ask me questions about where I have been.	Tell her to mind her own business!	She might think I'm being rude and not be my friend anymore.	3	5
	Be honest and tell her why I have been out of school.	I'm scared she will tease me, but she might be understanding and kind.	7	5
	Give her a brief answer and change the subject—say, "I've been scared about school, but I'm getting better now."	She might accept this, as I've given her an answer and hopefully she will be eager to talk about other things.	8	7
	Say that my grandma was ill.	She might not believe me, and I would feel bad for lying.	6	4

FIGURE 10.3. Laura's Problem-Solving Worksheet.

Holly did ask her another question, but then was happy to talk about other things.

Other Considerations

Support from the School

The parent and school working together are often crucial for a successful outcome. Some schools are more experienced at supporting children who refuse to attend than others. If parents feel that a particular teacher is not being as supportive as they had hoped, it may be helpful to encourage them to involve other staff members, as appropriate. There are often other personnel in school who are specifically responsible for children's special needs, as mentioned previously, who may be more experienced in these matters and can serve as a useful resource. Similarly, those responsible for overseeing school attendance (e.g., in the United Kingdom, education welfare officers [EWOs]) usually have a wealth of experience in dealing with school refusal and are often well versed in the principles of exposure. In our experience, if parents show a commitment to improving their child's school attendance, school personnel tend to be very receptive to supporting an appropriate program of reintegration. A good starting point is for parents to request a school meeting to discuss their concerns. Bringing along any material they have completed with you is a good way of showing the school staff what they are already doing to help resolve the problem and will also help to educate teaching staff about what kinds of strategies are likely to work.

Working with school personnel also allows parents to raise any concerns about learning that they and/or the child has identified that may be maintaining their child's nonattendance.

Limit Setting at Home

Inevitably, a child who is struggling to attend school will be spending many extra hours at home. If left to their own devices, most children will choose to engage in their favorite activities at these times, which might include playing computer games, watching TV, playing outside, or playing with toys. They are also likely to spend much more time with a parent, possibly engaging in enjoyable activities together. These activities can themselves be reinforcing for a child and maintain the child's school refusal difficulties further. It is thus important that you talk to parents about limit setting at home during the school day. It is important that there is a general expectation that the child will engage in school-related activities at this time, including formal work, but this might also include reading, watching an educational program on TV, visiting the library, or doing some research on the computer. We recommend that you encourage parents to limit (noneducational) computer and game time or ban them completely during school hours. This can be very difficult for parents to enforce because it requires a great deal of supervision on their part. However, it is likely to result in a marked increase in the child's motivation to reengage in school, as he or she is very likely to begin to view staying home as unstimulating and "boring" rather than "fun."

Distinguishing between Anxiety and Oppositional Behavior

As noted earlier, school refusal is not always associated with high levels of anxiety. Sometimes, it can be the result of significant oppositional behavior. A robust assessment will allow you to disentangle the two and to decide if clinically significant anxiety is driving the school refusal or not. We would recommend that you exercise caution in embarking on a program of parent-led CBT with a child who is refusing school who exhibits marked oppositional behavior and would certainly recommend that you read Chapter 11 for guidance.

Bullying

Children who refuse to attend school have sometimes been victims of bullying by their peers. Bullying should be recognized by school personnel and appropriate action must be taken. Working directly with parents will enable you to support them in talking to school personnel about a problem with bullying, which may be challenging and often anxiety-provoking for them. Nevertheless, it is important to convey that the responsibility lies with the school and not the child to address and resolve the issue.

Alongside action from the school, you may wish to consider with parents whether there are any strategies that the child could use in school to either alleviate the problem or to simply give the child some sense of control. Parents can work with the child using problem solving (Chapter 7 and "Problem Solving" on p. 168) to consider possible strategies and responses that the child may wish to try.

Home Tutoring/Changing Schools

Some parents believe that changing schools will resolve a school refusal problem. Not all families will have this option open to them, but working directly with parents is advantageous in that it allows you to have a thoughtful and frank discussion about changing schools and/or using home tutoring, should the parent raise one or both possibilities. In our experience, changing schools does not always lead to resolution of the anxiety problems, unless there is a clear rationale and the advantages outweigh the disadvantages. It may be advantageous when a child is struggling with the workload and is planning to enroll in a school that is better able to support him or her academically. If another child is specifically targeting the child with school refusal (but the child has not experienced similar difficulties in the past) and the school has not been able to successfully address this issue, it is possible that changing to a new school would resolve the issue.

There are, of course, a number of disadvantages to changing school, which include having to make new friends and get used to a new school environment. In general, we would recommend that parents try to work with the child and school to resolve any issues in the first instance. Parents may need a great deal of support from you to do so, in order to tolerate their child's high levels of distress until the situation improves. However, successfully resolving difficulties within the school can give children and parents a great deal of confidence in their ability to overcome challenges and will stand them in good stead for overcoming any future difficulties that may arise.

Similar considerations must be taken in to account when making a decision about home tutoring. In some cases, when a child's anxiety is extremely high, home tutoring can usefully form an initial part of an exposure plan for reintegration. In these cases, a child may first receive tutoring in the home, and then in the school setting, enabling the child to begin to attend classes alongside the individual tutoring. Home tutoring can be useful if it allows the child to keep up with work, despite being absent, preventing further anxieties about getting behind academically. If home tutoring is provided, careful thought and planning are required to ensure success, and it is crucial that parents able to convey a clear message to the child that home tutoring is a first step toward school attendance and not a long-term solution.

TAKE-HOME MESSAGES

✓ School refusal can be a result of high levels of anxiety, particularly social and separation anxiety.

✓ There is evidence that parents can use CBT to improve their child's school attendance.

✓ CBT strategies can be easily adapted to address school refusal issues.

✓ Graded exposure is likely to be the most important component of a CBT intervention for school refusal.

✓ Working directly with parents is advantageous because parents can liaise effectively with teachers and can work with their child to increase his or her motivation to achieve the goal.

CHAPTER 11

Treating Child Anxiety within Challenging Contexts

From training and supervising clinicians, as well as our own clinical work, we are aware that there are various contexts that can cause concerns about using a brief parent-led approach for treating child anxiety disorders. In this chapter, we focus on four of the most common contexts that create challenges in this work: when parents also have an anxiety disorder, or when children have behavioral problems, low mood, or limited social skills. We first consider what is known about each potential context in the research literature before making recommendations for overcoming it.

Parental Anxiety Disorders

What Does the Evidence Tell Us?

Are Parents of Children with Anxiety Disorders Also Likely to Be Highly Anxious?

It is well established that anxiety often runs in families (e.g., Eley et al., 2003). We conducted diagnostic interviews with the parents of children with anxiety disorders referred to our clinic and found that almost 70% of the mothers also met diagnostic criteria for an anxiety disorder, which was significantly different from the rates among mothers of nonanxious children (Cooper, Fearn, Willetts, Seabrook, & Parkinson, 2006). Interestingly, the rate of current anxiety disorders among fathers was not significantly elevated compared to the nonanxious comparison group, although fathers did have an inflated rate of lifetime anxiety disorders. Since that report we have found somewhat lower rates of anxiety disorders in mothers in our clinic, averaging around 50% (Creswell et al., 2015), but it remains clear that anxiety disorders are common among parents (particularly mothers) of children with anxiety disorders who present for treatment. The fact that anxiety disorders are more common among mothers than fathers is hardly surprising, given that anxiety disorders are more common among adult females than males (Bruce et al., 2008).

Does Parental Anxiety Disorder Affect Children's Treatment Outcomes?

A variety of approaches have been used to examine the association between parental anxiety and child anxiety treatment outcomes, and overall the findings are not entirely consistent. However, when the studies used a diagnostic interview with parents (rather than self-report symptom questionnaires), a more consistent picture appears in which the number of children who recover from treatment is about half what would otherwise be expected when their parents also have a current anxiety disorder (Bodden et al., 2008; Hudson et al., 2013). Few studies have examined this issue when CBT is delivered via parents; however, we found a similar pattern in one small study (Creswell, Willetts, Murray, Singhal, & Cooper, 2008) and also found that higher self-reported parent anxiety (but not depression or stress) symptoms were associated with poorer child outcomes in another (Creswell, Hentges, et al., 2010).

An obvious implication of these studies is that parents might need treatment for their own anxiety disorders; however, when this possibility has been examined, findings have been inconsistent (Cobham, Dadds, & Spence, 1998; Hudson et al., 2013; Creswell et al., 2015). All in all, there is no clear evidence that improving parental anxiety benefits child treatment outcomes; however, the studies were all limited by fairly brief treatments for parental anxiety disorders that brought about fairly low levels of change in parental anxiety. Another explanation for the relatively poor outcomes for children with anxiety disorders whose parents have an anxiety disorder is that particular parental responses (that are more common among highly anxious parents) may reinforce child anxiety disorders, and, as such, be an obstacle to good child treatment outcomes. By observing interactions in the lab between primary caregiving mothers and their anxious children, we have found that the mothers who had an anxiety disorder had more negative expectations of their child, expressed more anxiety, and were more intrusive in their interactions, particularly when the child was visibly stressed by the task (Creswell et al., 2013). There was also evidence to suggest that the more anxious mothers felt during the task, the more negative the interaction. These findings suggest that parents of children with anxiety disorders who also have an anxiety disorder themselves may find it hard to tolerate their child's distress, making it difficult for them to support their child in effective exposure treatment.

Despite these observational findings, it remains unclear exactly what needs to happen to optimize children's outcomes. Much of the lack of clarity could stem from the reciprocal nature of the relationships between children's and parents' responses. For example, particular parental responses may be elicited among anxious parents only if their child is also anxious (e.g., Hirshfeld, Biederman, Brody, Faraone, & Rosenbaum, 1997). We recently supplemented individual child CBT with an intervention that aimed to target potentially anxiety-promoting aspects of the mother–child interaction. We found fairly limited differences in how parents and their children interacted after the intervention, compared to child CBT plus a control intervention (Creswell et al., 2015), which may well reflect the fact that parental behaviors will change in response to their child's response to treatment (e.g., Silverman, Kurtines, Jaccard, & Pina, 2009). Treatment recovery rates did not differ following CBT plus this adjunct intervention, compared to those among children who received CBT plus a control intervention—although notably, there were some longer-term differences in child anxiety severity that appeared to be associated with an overall cost–benefit from delivering CBT with the parent–child interaction- focused treatment.

What Are the Implications for a Parent-Focused Approach?

It has been suggested that parental anxiety disorders may pose a particular difficulty when parents are relied upon to deliver the treatment (e.g., Chavira et al., 2014). It is also possible, of course, that this sort of treatment might be particularly helpful if it can successfully address any issues that might otherwise make it difficult for parents to support their child's recovery. We recently ran a small trial to examine whether supplementing a brief parent-led approach with strategies to help parents increase their tolerance of their child's negative emotions would improve child treatment outcomes in the context of high parental anxiety. We found no added benefit to adding these additional strategies; however, notably, across both the standard and adapted treatment arms, treatment outcomes were good (55–60% diagnosis free) and similar to outcomes achieved from this low-intensity intervention (and more intensive CBT interventions) with nonselected parents of children with anxiety disorders (Hiller et al., 2016). These findings suggest that a brief parent-delivered intervention is a feasible treatment for child anxiety disorders, even in the context of high parental anxiety. Furthermore, we found that self-reported parental anxiety was significantly reduced in both treatment arms. In this particular study parents had about an hour more therapist time than we typically provide. Whether this led to better outcomes than might otherwise be expected remains unclear, but allowing more time in the context of high parental anxiety may make sense, given the suggestion that reduced treatment outcomes among children with anxiety disorders who have highly anxious parents might be explained by characteristics of general family functioning or family stress (e.g., Schleider, Patel, Krumholz, Chorpita, & Weisz, 2015). As such, parents may require a bit more time and support in putting the treatment into place within these challenging contexts.

Recommendations for Working in the Context of Parental Anxiety Disorder

Do Offer This Treatment

On the basis of the evidence presented above and our clinical experience, we strongly suggest that therapists do *not* put off offering a parent-focused approach in the context of parental anxiety disorder. Brief parent-focused treatment can be effective for children with anxiety disorders even in the context of high parental anxiety, and may also lead to reductions in parental anxiety. However, as when working with any parent, it is important to establish and monitor whether the parents are able to make a commitment to engaging with the treatment. For example, are they are able to prioritize it, given the other challenges they are facing? Are they motivated to do so? In establishing this point, it is essential to distinguish between, for example, lack of motivation and lack of confidence. Many parents are concerned that they won't be able to help their child, and we have found that high parental anxiety is associated with a particular lack of perceived control over their child's responses (e.g., Wheatcroft & Creswell, 2007). This finding is understandable, given the struggles they have had that led them to seek help; however, a parent-led approach can increase parents' confidence in their ability to support their child—an important treatment outcome.

Keep Treatment on Track

Therapists also need to take care to ensure that the treatment isn't pulled off track by a focus on the parents' own difficulties. It is essential to understand the difficulties that parents face and to acknowledge the challenges posed. However, it is also important not to assume that they will interfere with treatment for the child and to keep the focus on helping the child overcome his or her difficulties. Setting a clear agenda at the start of each session is important to achieve this focus. As we have noted above, allowing a bit more therapist time to help support parents in problem-solving how to put the principles in place, given the other challenges they face, might be useful. However, if a parent seems to need a significant amount of time to discuss his or her own difficulties with anxiety, then it is important to recognize this need and to help the parent seek support in his or her own right. Similarly, if parental anxiety is a response to living in particularly challenging circumstances (e.g., parental relationship breakdown), then it is essential to establish whether these circumstances will make it more difficult for the parent to put the strategies in this book in place in an environment that supports positive changes for the child. Sometimes it is just not the right time to embark on this approach. Families need to make an informed choice about the timing on the basis of information about what treatment involves and the degree of commitment that is required from them.

Working in the Context of Other Parental Mental Health Difficulties

Although we have focused here on parental anxiety disorders, of course parents will also present with other mental health problems. In our view, these same basic principles apply in deciding with the parent whether this is a useful approach to take—that is: Is the parent able to make a commitment to the treatment? Is the parent motivated to engage in the treatment? Will the parent be able to foster an environment that promotes his or her child's recovery? If the parent is experiencing significant mental health problems, such as moderate to severe depression, we suggest referring the parent to appropriate adult services for his or her own treatment. Some parents engage in their own therapy before working on their child's anxiety, or they may choose to get treatment for themselves alongside the child-focused treatment. Making this decision is best based on whichever choice is likely to be the most practical and achievable for the family.

Child Behavior Problems

What Does the Evidence Tell Us?

Do Children with Anxiety Disorders Often Have Comorbid Behavior Problems?

Whereas many anxious children do not present with overt behavior difficulties and may present as quiet, withdrawn, and quite compliant, particularly at school, some children will exhibit difficult behaviors (e.g., crying, shouting, or refusing to go somewhere or do something) in response to their specific anxiety disorder. For example, a child with significant separation anxiety may show "difficult" behaviors when it is time to be separated from the caregiver, such as on a Monday morning before school. In this example, the child expresses his or her fears behaviorally, often in an attempt to avoid the feared situation. It is important to help parents notice patterns when these sorts of behaviors occur. If they are mainly seen before or during anxiety-provoking situations, it is likely that they are an anxiety symptom rather than a comorbid behavior problem. Whereas if they tend to occur when a child can't do or have what he or she wants, then they may reflect more oppositional difficulties that are comorbid with anxiety. Indeed, a proportion of children (approximately 6%; Waite & Creswell, 2014) with anxiety disorders also experience comorbid behavior problems such as aggressive or oppositional behavior.

Do Comorbid Behavior Problems Affect Children's Treatment Outcomes?

A number of studies that have examined predictors of outcome from CBT for childhood anxiety problems have shown that children with comorbid behavior difficulties do not do as well in treatment as anxious children who don't have these problems. For example, in a large, international multisite study, Hudson et al. (2013, 2015) found that comorbid externalizing disorders significantly predicted poorer treatment outcomes for children with anxiety immediately after treatment and later at follow-up, even after accounting for pretreatment anxiety severity. However, comorbid externalizing difficulties seemed to have a less negative impact on outcomes at the follow-up time point, suggesting that children with comorbid behavioral disorders may take longer to improve. On the other hand, it has also been shown that behavior problems do not improve following anxiety treatment (Rapee et al., 2013), suggesting that these problems may need intervention in their own right.

There has been very little evaluation of whether the co-occurrence of behavior problems is associated with relatively poor outcomes following parent-led CBT for child anxiety disorders specifically. However, in a recent study, we did not find that comorbid behavior disorders negatively affected child treatment outcomes in a parent-led intervention (Thirlwall et al., 2016). Although further investigation is required, it may be that a parent-focused approach is well suited to managing anxiety disorders in the context of comorbid behavior problems because a number of the strategies that parents are putting in to place may also be helpful in managing challenging behavior (e.g., setting clear expectations and providing associated praise and rewards).

How Can Children's Treatment Outcomes Be Improved in the Context of Comorbid Behavior Problems?

Based on the currently available literature and the mixed findings, it is difficult to identify specific ways in which children's treatment outcomes could be improved when anxiety problems co-occur with behavior problems. On the basis of the findings that these children may not do as well in individual treatment as those without comorbid behavior problems, it could be hypothesized that providing an extra intervention aimed at the behavior difficulties would produce better outcomes. However, conversely similar improvements have been found in both anxiety and aggression in children who received either individual CBT for anxiety only or CBT for anxiety and aggression (Levy, Hunt, & Heriot, 2007). Furthermore, comorbid behavior problems did not affect outcomes for anxious children in a parent-led program (Thirlwall et al., 2016). Therefore, there is reason to believe that additional behavior interventions are not always needed in these circumstances.

Recommendations for Working in the Context of Comorbid Child Behavior Problems

Do Offer This Treatment If Anxiety Is the Primary Problem

If a child is experiencing both anxiety difficulties and behavior problems, it is important to first establish which is the primary problem (see Chapter 2). If anxiety is the main difficulty, then we recommend that this program is applied and the behavior problems are monitored throughout treatment. It will also be important to develop with parents a shared understanding of the main problems (see Chapters 2 and 3) and to establish shared goals for treatment, being clear that the behavior problems will not be the focus of the anxiety intervention (see end of Chapter 2). Sometimes we have observed that as the anxiety difficulties improve, some of the behavior difficulties seem more manageable. If any significant behavior difficulties remain after the anxiety treatment, we suggest you discuss these with parents and refer them to the appropriate interventions.

If it is the case that behavior difficulties are causing the most difficulties for the family and anxiety is secondary, we recommend that the appropriate treatment for the behavior difficulties first be sought. Once the behavior problems have improved, any anxiety difficulties can be addressed.

Child Mood Disorders

What Does the Evidence Tell Us?

Do Children with Anxiety Disorders Often Have Comorbid Mood Disorders?

Only a small proportion of preadolescent children with anxiety also experience mood problems, with estimates of approximately 1% of children with anxiety having a concurrent mood disorder (e.g., Waite & Creswell, 2015).

Do Comorbid Mood Disorders Affect Children's Anxiety Treatment Outcomes?

The findings are mixed, but generally it seems that children with comorbid mood disorders show poorer outcomes from CBT for anxiety disorders. Some studies have shown that children with comorbid mood disorders such as depression respond well to anxiety-focused treatment, and that comorbid mood disorders are not associated with treatment outcomes (Kendall, Aschenbrand, & Hudson, 2003; Kendall et al., 1997). However, other studies have found a significant association between comorbid mood problems and treatment outcomes. For example, Berman, Weems, Silverman, and Kurtines (2000) found that those children with comorbid depression were more likely to be "treatment failures" following an exposure-based treatment. In addition, the treatment failure group was much more likely than the treatment success group to have higher self-rated scores for low mood. Similarly, in a large multisite study, Hudson et al. (2015) found that comorbid mood disorders significantly predicted poorer outcomes for children after treatment and at a later point at follow-up. Rapee (2003) reported similar findings, but also noted that children with comorbid depression did report improved mood following anxiety-focused CBT.

Just as for behavioral problems, there has been very little evaluation of whether comorbid mood disorders are associated with poor outcomes following parent-led CBT for child anxiety disorders specifically. However, we have recently found that comorbid mood disorders were not associated with treatment outcome either immediately after treatment or 6 months later (Thirlwall et al., 2016). Further investigation is required, but for now the findings suggest that it is reasonable to offer a parent-led approach in the context of comorbid mood disorders when anxiety is the primary problem.

How Can Children's Treatment Outcomes Be Improved in the Context of Comorbid Mood Disorders?

A number of studies have shown that interventions for anxiety in children can also lead to reductions in depressive symptoms (e.g., Kendall, Hudson, Gosch, Flannery-Schroeder, & Suveg, 2008; Kendall, Safford, Flannery-Schroeder, & Webb, 2004; Manassis et al., 2002), which may reflect the overlap in content between CBT for anxiety and depression and the overlap in the two disorders in children (Laurent & Ettelson, 2001). However, we are not aware of any studies that have directly examined additional treatment of comorbid low mood in the context of anxiety disorders in this age group, so the benefits of this remain unclear.

Recommendations for Working in the Context of Comorbid Child Mood Disorders

Do Offer This Treatment If Anxiety Is the Primary Problem

As highlighted in the behavior difficulties section, a thorough assessment is necessary to determine whether anxiety or mood disorders are the primary problem (see Chapter 2). If mood disorders are the primary problem, there are two options. The first option is to offer an intervention that deals with both anxiety and mood disorders simultaneously. Kendall, Kortlander, Chansky and Brady, (1992) and Berman et al. (2000) suggest targeting both depression and anxiety when these are comorbid. The second option would be to offer or refer the child for a mood disorder intervention before working on the anxiety difficulties. In these circumstances, sharing findings from the assessment with the family will be important to inform the choice of treatment option.

If anxiety is the primary problem, we recommend that this treatment be offered for the anxiety and that the child's mood be monitored throughout. Monitoring the child's mood will indicate whether the intervention has also had a positive impact on the mood disorder or if further input to target mood is required.

Social Skills Deficits

What Does the Evidence Tell Us?

Do Children with Anxiety Disorders Exhibit Social Skills Deficits?

Social skills deficits have been implicated in models of social anxiety disorder in children (e.g., Rapee & Spence, 2004), and specific treatments for social anxiety disorder in children often include a substantial focus on improving children's social skills (e.g., Beidel & Turner, 2007; Spence, Donovan, & Brechman-Toussaint, 2000). This approach is in contrast to adult models of social anxiety disorder that typically highlight the importance of beliefs about low social competence among people with social anxiety disorder in the absence of actual deficits (e.g., Clark & Wells, 1995; Rapee & Heimberg, 1997). Whereas studies that rely on self-report have suggested that there may be perceived social skills deficits among adults with social anxiety disorder (e.g., Stopa & Clark, 1993), observational studies have produced more mixed results (e.g., Thompson & Rapee, 2002; Rapee & Lim, 1992), and treatments that target cognitive distortions, rather than actual social skills deficits, have produced excellent results (e.g., Clark et al., 2003). Despite these findings with adults, it has been suggested that early social skills deficits may put children at risk of social anxiety disorder (Rapee & Spence, 2004). In support of this suggestion, Spence, Donovan and Brechman-Toussaint (1999) found that children with social anxiety rated themselves as less socially skilled than nonanxious children, and this was supported by both parental report and direct behavioral observation. However, it is possible that the social skills "deficits" that were observed (i.e., length of response to another child, the number of peer interactions, and the number of initiations made by the child) may have reflected children's increased inhibition in social encounters due to feeling anxious. Consistent with this suggestion, Cartwright-Hatton, Hodges, and Porter (2003) found no evidence of poor social skills among 8- to 11-year-old children with high levels of social anxiety when they engaged in a public speaking task, although these children were more "concerned" about their social skills than low socially anxious children. In a subsequent study, Cartwright-Hatton, Tschernitz, and Gomersall (2005) again found no difference between the social skills of socially anxious children in comparison to a nonanxious control group, but did find significant differences in self-reported social skills. On the basis of these findings, Cartwright-Hatton et al. warned that social skills training may reinforce the idea that socially anxious children are lacking social skills, enhancing cognitive distortions about their social performance and increasing their anxiety levels.

Taken together, it would be reasonable to conclude from the findings that a deficit in social skills is not necessarily a key feature of social anxiety in children, and, in fact, the majority of children with social anxiety are likely to have adequate social skills. However, they are likely to perceive their performance in social interaction negatively. It also remains possible that a subgroup of children with anxiety disorders, particularly social anxiety disorder, may experience comorbid difficulties with social skills. For example, we found that children with social anxiety disorder were three times more likely to score above clinical cutoffs (8.8%) than children with other anxiety disorders (2.1%) on the basis of a screening questionnaire for social communication difficulties that covers reciprocal social interaction, communication, and restricted and repetitive behaviors (Halls, Cooper, & Creswell, 2015). These findings suggest that a proportion of children with social anxiety disorder might benefit from a specific focus on developing their social skills.

Do Social Skills Deficits Affect Children's Treatment Outcomes?

Very few studies have examined this particular issue. Notably higher ratings (by the index child) of friendship quality with a close friend have been found to be associated with better treatment outcomes for anxious children (Baker & Hudson, 2013). However, friendship quality, as rated by the index child's friend, was not significantly associated with treatment outcome. As such, it remains unclear whether the index child's ability to form good friendships (which is likely to be associated with the quality of his or her social skills) influenced outcome, or whether the findings reflected the child's distorted perceptions of these friendships. A further study looked more directly at social communication by examining the association between autistic symptomology (based on parent-reported reciprocal social behavior and behavioral observations) and treatment outcome for childhood anxiety following a family-based versus individual CBT treatment (Puleo & Kendall, 2011). Higher levels of autistic symptomology were associated with poorer outcomes for individual CBT but not for family-based CBT. These findings suggest that working with family members of anxious children with comorbid social communication difficulties may be particularly important to help engage these children in treatment and to promote generalization of treatment gains through home-based tasks.

Recommendations for Working in the Context of Social Skills Deficits

Do Offer This Treatment If Anxiety Is the Primary Problem (Tentatively)

Given that a proportion of children with anxiety disorders (particularly those with social anxiety disorder) may experience difficulties with social skills or communication, it is important to assess (1) whether the child has social skills deficits *or* whether the child perceives these deficits but actually functions well in social interactions; and (2) how any social skills deficits contribute to the difficulties with anxiety. A child's social skills can be assessed by observation, clinical interview, and/or the use of standardized questionnaire measures (e.g., Social Skills Questionnaire; Spence, 1995). However, it is important to not rely solely on self-report, given the possibility of biased perceptions of one's own social skills. Information from teachers as well as parents, as well as observational assessments, can often be enormously helpful in fully understanding how the child functions socially in a variety of settings.

If there is clear evidence that a child has social skills difficulties and that these are contributing to the child's difficulties with anxiety, it is important to monitor progress in treatment in order to establish whether a specific focus on these difficulties is required. Indeed, effective treatments that have a particular focus on developing social skills have been developed for children with anxiety disorders in the context of ASD. For example, Wood et al. (2009) enhanced standard CBT with child, parent, and teacher modules to address poor social skills (through teaching and social coaching) and school-based problems (including peer "buddy" and mentoring programs).

If the child has a negative perception of his or her social skills, but there is no evidence of social skills deficits, these negative expectations can be worked on by parents, using the strategies outlined earlier in the book (e.g., encouraging "have a go" thinking, Chapter 5; helping children to face their fears, Chapter 6).

TAKE-HOME MESSAGES

✓ Parent-led CBT for childhood anxiety disorders may be effective in challenging contexts.

✓ Careful assessment and monitoring of comorbid difficulties are important to establish whether these difficulties remit with treatment or require intervention in their own right.

References

Aktar, E., Majdandžić, M., de Vente, W., & Bögels, S. M. (2013). The interplay between expressed parental anxiety and infant behavioural inhibition predicts infant avoidance in a social referencing paradigm. *Journal of Child Psychology and Psychiatry, 54,* 144–156.

Alfano, C. A., Beidel, D. C., & Turner, S. M. (2002). Cognition in childhood anxiety: Conceptual, methodological, and developmental issues. *Clinical Psychology Review, 22,* 1209–1238.

Alfano, C. A., Ginsburg, G. S., & Kingery, J. N. (2007). Sleep-related problems among children and adolescents with anxiety disorders. *Journal of the American Academy of Child and Adolescent Psychiatry, 46,* 224–232.

Alfano, C. A., & Mellman, T. A. (2010). Sleep in anxiety disorders. In J. W. Winkelman & D. T. Plante (Eds.), *Foundations of psychiatric sleep medicine* (pp. 286–297). New York: Cambridge University Press.

Alfano, C. A., Pina, A. A., Zerr, A. A., & Villalta, I. K. (2010). Pre-sleep arousal and sleep problems of anxiety-disordered youth. *Child Psychiatry and Human Development, 41,* 156–167.

Alkozei, A., Cooper, P. J., & Creswell, C. (2014). Emotional reasoning and anxiety sensitivity: Associations with social anxiety disorder in childhood. *Journal of Affective Disorders, 152,* 219–228.

Allen, J. L., Rapee, R. M., & Sandberg, S. (2008). Severe life events and chronic adversities as antecedents to anxiety in children: A matched control study. *Journal of Abnormal Child Psychology, 36,* 1047–1056.

American Psychiatric Association. (2013). *Diagnostic and statistical manual of mental disorders* (5th ed.). Arlington, VA: Author.

Amir, N., Beard, C., & Bower, E. (2005). Interpretation bias and social anxiety. *Cognitive Therapy and Research, 29,* 433–443.

Baker, J., & Hudson, J. (2013). Friendship quality predicts treatment outcome in children with anxiety disorders. *Behaviour Research and Therapy, 51,* 31–36.

Bar-Haim, Y., Lamy, D., Pergamin, L., Bakermans-Kranenburg, M. J., & van IJzendoorn, M. H. (2007). Threat-related attentional bias in anxious and nonanxious individuals: A meta-analytic study. *Psychological Bulletin, 133*, 1–24.

Barrett, P. M., Dadds, M. R., & Rapee, R. M. (1996). Family treatment of childhood anxiety: A controlled trial. *Journal of Consulting and Clinical Psychology,
64*, 333–342.

Beck, A. T., & Clark, D. A. (1997). An information processing model of anxiety: Automatic and strategic processes. *Behaviour Research and Therapy, 35*,
49–58.

Beidel, D. C., & Turner, S. M. (1997). At risk for anxiety: I. Psychopathology in
the offspring of anxious parents. *Journal of the American Academy of Child and
Adolescent Psychiatry, 36*, 918–924.

Beidel, D. C., & Turner, S. M. (2007). *Shy children, phobic adults: Nature and treatment of social anxiety disorder* (2nd ed.). Washington, DC: American Psychological Association

Berg, I., Nichols, K., & Pritchard, C. (1969). School phobia—its classification and
relationship to dependency. *Journal of Child Psychology and Psychiatry, 10*,
123–141.

Berman, S. L., Weems, C. F., Silverman, W. K., & Kurtines, W. M. (2000). Predictors of outcome in exposure-based cognitive and behavioral treatments for
phobic and anxiety disorders in children. *Behavior Therapy, 31*, 713–731.

Bickman, L., Kelley, S. D., Breda, C., de Andrade, A. R., & Riemer, M. (2011).
Effects of routine feedback to clinicians on mental health outcomes of youths:
Results of a randomized trial. *Psychiatric Services, 62*, 1423–1429.

Bijttebier, P., Vasey, M. W., & Braet, C. (2003). The information-processing paradigm: A valuable framework for clinical child and adolescent psychology.
Journal of Clinical Child and Adolescent Psychology, 32, 2–9.

Bishop, D. (2003). *The Children's Communication Checklist, version 2 (CCC-2)*.
London: Pearson

Blagg, N. (1987). *School phobia and its management*. London: Croom Helm.

Blagg, N., & Yule, W. (1984). The behavioural treatment of school refusal—a com-
parative study. *Behaviour Research and Therapy, 22*, 119–127.

Bodden, D. H., Bögels, S. M., Nauta, M. H., De Haan, E., Ringrose, J., Appel-
boom, C., et al. (2008). Child versus family cognitive-behavioral therapy in
clinically anxious youth: An efficacy and partial effectiveness study. *Journal
of the American Academy of Child and Adolescent Psychiatry, 47*, 1384–1394.

Bouchard, S., Mendlowitz, S. L., Coles, M. E., & Franklin, M. (2005). Considerations in the use of exposure with children. *Cognitive and Behavioral Practice,
11*, 56–65.

Briggs-Gowan, M. J., Carter, A. S., & Schwab-Stone, M. (1996). Discrepancies
among mother, child, and teacher reports: Examining the contributions of
maternal depression and anxiety. *Journal of Abnormal Child Psychology, 24*,
749–765.

Brown, A., Thirlwall, K., & Creswell, C. (2016). *Parent-delivered guided CBT bibliotherapy for children with anxiety: Outcomes at four-year follow-up*. Manuscript submitted for publication.

Bruce, S. E., Yonkers, K. A., Otto, M. W., Eisen, J. L., Weisberg, R. B., Pagano, M., et al. (2008). Influence of psychiatric comorbidity on recovery and recurrence in generalized anxiety disorder, social phobia, and panic disorder: A 12-year prospective study. *Focus, 6,* 539–548.

Bruni, O., Ottaviano, S., Guidetti, V., Romoli, M., Innocenzi, M., Cortesi, F., et al. (1997). The Sleep Disturbance Scale for Children (SDSC): Construction and validation of an instrument to evaluate sleep disturbances in childhood and adolescence. *Journal of Sleep Research, 5,* 251–261.

Caporino, N. E., Brodman, D. M., Kendall, P. C., Albano, A. M., Sherrill, J., Piacentini, J., et al. (2013). Defining treatment response and remission in child anxiety: Signal detection analysis using the pediatric anxiety rating scale. *Journal of the American Academy of Child and Adolescent Psychiatry, 52,* 57–67.

Capps, L., Sigman, M., Sena, R., Heoker, B., & Whalen, C. (1996). Fear, anxiety and perceived control in children of agoraphobic parents. *Journal of Child Psychology and Psychiatry, 37,* 445–452.

Cartwright-Hatton, S., Hodges, L., & Porter, J. (2003). Social anxiety in childhood: The relationship with self and observer rated social skills. *Journal of Child Psychology and Psychiatry, 44,* 737–742.

Cartwright-Hatton, S., McNally, D., Field, A. P., Rust, S., Laskey, B., Dixon, C., et al. (2011). A new parenting-based group intervention for young anxious children: Results of a randomized controlled trial. *Journal of the American Academy of Child and Adolescent Psychiatry, 50,* 242–251.

Cartwright-Hatton, S., Tschernitz, N., & Gomersall, H. (2005). Social anxiety in children: Social skills deficit or cognitive distortion? *Behaviour Research and Therapy, 43,* 131–141.

Chan, C. W., Richardson, A., & Richardson, J. (2011). Managing symptoms in patients with advanced lung cancer during radiotherapy: Results of a psychoeducational randomized controlled trial. *Journal of Pain and Symptom Management, 41,* 347–357.

Chavira, D. A., Drahota, A., Garland, A. F., Roesch, S., Garcia, M., & Stein, M. B. (2014). Feasibility of two modes of treatment delivery for child anxiety in primary care. *Behaviour Research and Therapy, 60,* 60–66.

Chorpita, B. F., & Barlow, D. H. (1998). The development of anxiety: The role of control in the early environment. *Psychological Bulletin, 124,* 3–21.

Chorpita, B. F., Yim, L., Moffitt, C., Umemoto, L. A., & Francis, S. E. (2000). Assessment of symptoms of DSM-IV anxiety and depression in children: A revised child anxiety and depression scale. *Behaviour Research and Therapy, 38,* 835–855.

Clark, D. M., Ehlers, A., McManus, F., Hackmann, A., Fennell, M., Campbell, H., et al. (2003). Cognitive therapy versus fluoxetine in generalized social phobia: A randomized placebo-controlled trial. *Journal of Consulting and Clinical Psychology, 71,* 1058–1067.

Clark, D. M., & Wells, A. (1995). A cognitive model of social phobia. In G. Heimberg, M. Liebovitz, D. Hope, & F. Scheier (Eds.), *Social phobia: Diagnosis, assessment, and treatment* (pp. 69–93). New York: Guilford Press.

Clementi, M. A., & Alfano, C. A. (2014). Targeted behavioral therapy for childhood generalized anxiety disorder: A time-series analysis of changes in anxiety and sleep. *Journal of Anxiety Disorders, 28,* 215–222.

Cobham, V. E. (2012). Do anxiety-disordered children need to come into the clinic for efficacious treatment? *Journal of Consulting and Clinical Psychology, 80,* 465–476.

Cobham, V. E., Dadds, M. R., & Spence, S. H. (1998). The role of parental anxiety in the treatment of childhood anxiety. *Journal of Consulting and Clinical Psychology, 66,* 893–905.

Cooper, P. J., Fearn, V., Willetts, L., Seabrook, H., & Parkinson, M. (2006). Affective disorder in the parents of a clinic sample of children with anxiety disorders. *Journal of Affective Disorders, 93,* 205–212.

Craske, M. G., Kircanski, K., Zelikowsky, M., Mystkowski, J., Chowdhury, N., & Baker, A. (2008). Optimizing inhibitory learning during exposure therapy. *Behaviour Research and Therapy, 46,* 5–27.

Craske, M. G., Treanor, M., Conway, C. C., Zbozinek, T., & Vervliet, B. (2014). Maximizing exposure therapy: An inhibitory learning approach. *Behaviour Research and Therapy, 58,* 10–23.

Crawley, S. A., Kendall, P. C., Benjamin, C. L., Brodman, D. M., Wei, C., Beidas, R. S., et al. (2013). Brief cognitive-behavioral therapy for anxious youth: Feasibility and initial outcomes. *Cognitive and Behavioral Practice, 20,* 123–133.

Creswell, C., Apetroaia, A., Murray, L., & Cooper, P. (2013). Cognitive, affective, and behavioral characteristics of mothers with anxiety disorders in the context of child anxiety disorder. *Journal of Abnormal Psychology, 122,* 26–38.

Creswell, C., Cooper, P., & Murray, L. (2010). Intergenerational transmission of anxious information processing biases. In J. Hadwin & A. Field (Eds.), *Information processing biases and anxiety: A developmental perspective* (pp. 279–296). Chichester, UK: Wiley.

Creswell, C., Cruddace, S., Gerry, S., Gitau, R., McIntosh, E., Mollison, J., et al. (2015). Treatment of childhood anxiety disorder in the context of maternal anxiety disorder: A randomised controlled trial and economic analysis. *Health Technology Assessment, 19,* 1–184.

Creswell, C., Hentges, F., Parkinson, M., Sheffield, P., Willetts, L., & Cooper, P. (2010). Feasibility of guided cognitive behaviour therapy (CBT) self-help for childhood anxiety disorders in primary care. *Mental Health in Family Medicine, 7,* 49–57.

Creswell, C., Murray, L., & Cooper, P. (2014). Interpretation and expectation in childhood anxiety disorders: Age effects and social specificity. *Journal of Abnormal Child Psychology, 42,* 453–465.

Creswell, C., & O'Connor, T. G. (2011). Interpretation bias and anxiety in childhood: Stability, specificity and longitudinal associations. *Behavioural and Cognitive Psychotherapy, 39,* 191–204.

Creswell, C., O'Connor, T. G., & Brewin, C. R. (2008). The impact of parents' expectations on parenting behaviour: An experimental investigation. *Behavioural and Cognitive Psychotherapy, 36,* 483–490.

Creswell, C., Schniering, C. A., & Rapee, R. M. (2005). Threat interpretation in anxious children and their mothers: Comparison with nonclinical children and the effects of treatment. *Behaviour Research and Therapy, 43,* 1375–1381.

Creswell, C., & Willetts, L. (2007). *Overcoming your child's fears and worries: A self-help guide using cognitive-behavioural techniques.* London: Constable Robinson.

Creswell, C., Willetts, L., Murray, L., Singhal, M., & Cooper, P. (2008). Treatment of child anxiety: An exploratory study of the role of maternal anxiety and behaviours in treatment outcome. *Clinical Psychology and Psychotherapy, 15,* 38–44.

Davey, G. C. (1994). Worrying, social problem-solving abilities, and social problem-solving confidence. *Behaviour Research and Therapy, 32,* 327–330.

de Rosnay, M., Cooper, P. J., Tsigaras, N., & Murray, L. (2006). Transmission of social anxiety from mother to infant: An experimental study using a social referencing paradigm. *Behaviour Research and Therapy, 44,* 1165–1175.

de Ross, R. L., Gullone, E., & Chorpita, B. F. (2002). The Revised Child Anxiety and Depression Scale: A psychometric investigation with Australian youth. *Behaviour Change, 19,* 90–101.

de Wilde, A., & Rapee, R. M. (2008). Do controlling maternal behaviours increase state anxiety in children's responses to a social threat?: A pilot study. *Journal of Behavior Therapy and Experimental Psychiatry, 39,* 526–537.

Dinges, D. F., Pack, F., Williams, K., Gillen, K. A., Powell, J. W., Ott, G. E., et al. (1997). Cumulative sleepiness, mood disturbance and psychomotor vigilance performance decrements during a week of sleep restricted to 4–5 hours per night. *Sleep, 20,* 267–277.

Donker, T., Griffiths, K. M., Cuijpers, P., & Christensen, H. (2009). Psychoeducation for depression, anxiety and psychological distress: A meta-analysis. *BMC Medicine, 7,* 79.

Ebesutani, C., Bernstein, A., Nakamura, B. J., Chorpita, B. F., Weisz, J. R., & the Research Network on Youth Mental Health. (2010). A psychometric analysis of the Revised Child Anxiety And Depression Scale—Parent Version in a clinical sample. *Journal of Abnormal Child Psychology, 38,* 249–260.

Eley, T. C., Bolton, D., O'Connor, T. G., Perrin, S., Smith, P., & Plomin, R. (2003). A twin study of anxiety-related behaviours in pre-school children. *Journal of Child Psychology and Psychiatry, 44,* 945–960.

Eley, T. C., McAdams, T. A., Rijsdijk, F. V., Lichtenstein, P., Narusyte, J., Reiss, D., et al. (2015). The intergenerational transmission of anxiety: A children-of-twins study. *American Journal of Psychiatry, 172,* 630–637.

Espie, C. A. (2006). *Overcoming insomnia and sleep problems.* London: Robinson.

Essau, C. A., & Gabbidon, J. (2013). Epidemiology, comorbidity and mental health services utilization. In C. A. Essau & T. H. Ollendick (Eds.), *The Wiley–Blackwell handbook of the treatment of childhood and adolescent anxiety* (pp. 23–42). Chichester, UK: Wiley.

Evans, R., Thirlwall, K., Cooper, P., & Creswell, C. (in press). Using symptom and interference questionnaires to identify recovery among children with anxiety disorders. *Psychological Assessment.*

Field, A. P., & Lawson, J. (2003). Fear information and the development of fears during childhood: Effects on implicit fear responses and behavioural avoidance. *Behaviour Research and Therapy, 41,* 1277–1293.

Fivush, R. (1991). Gender and emotion in mother–child conversations about the past. *Journal of Narrative and Life History, 1,* 325–341.

Foa, E. B., & Kozak, M. J. (1986). Emotional processing of fear: Exposure to corrective information. *Psychological Bulletin, 99,* 20–35.

Fox, N. A., Nichols, K. E., Henderson, H. A., Rubin, K., Schmidt, L., Hamer, D., et al. (2005). Evidence for a gene–environment interaction in predicting behavioral inhibition in middle childhood. *Psychological Science, 16,* 921–926.

Gallant, P. (2013). "No worry allowed. Get out!": A case study tribute to the life and work of Michael White. *Contemporary Family Therapy, 35,* 29–40.

Gerull, F. C., & Rapee, R. M. (2002). Mother knows best: Effects of maternal modelling on the acquisition of fear and avoidance behaviour in toddlers. *Behaviour Research and Therapy, 40,* 279–287.

Goodman, R. (1997). The Strengths and Difficulties Questionnaire: A research note. *Journal of Child Psychology and Psychiatry, 38,* 581–586.

Gregory, A. M., & Eley, T. C. (2007). Genetic influences on anxiety in children: What we've learned and where we're heading. *Clinical Child and Family Psychology Review, 10,* 199–212.

Halls, G., Cooper, P. J., & Creswell, C. (2015). Social communication deficits: Specific associations with Social Anxiety Disorder. *Journal of Affective Disorders, 172,* 38–42.

Hamilton, D. I., & King, N. J. (1991). Reliability of a behavioral avoidance test for the assessment of dog phobic children. *Psychological Reports, 69,* 18.

Hedtke, K. A., Kendall, P. C., & Tiwari, S. (2009). Safety-seeking and coping behavior during exposure tasks with anxious youth. *Journal of Clinical Child and Adolescent Psychology, 38,* 1–15.

Hersov, L. A. (1960). Refusal to go to school. *Journal of Child Psychology and Psychiatry, 1,* 137–145.

Heyne, D., King, N. J., Tonge, B. J., Rollings, S., Young, D., Pritchard, M., et al. (2002). Evaluation of child therapy and caregiver training in the treatment of school refusal. *Journal of the American Academy of Child and Adolescent Psychiatry, 41,* 687–695.

Higa-McMillan, C. K., Francis, S. E., Rith-Najarian, L., & Chorpita, B. F. (2015). Evidence base update: 50 years of research on treatment for child and adolescent anxiety. *Journal of Clinical Child and Adolescent Psychology, 45*(2), 91–113.

Hiller, R., Apetroaia, A., Clarke, K., Hughes, Z., Orchard, F., Parkinson, M., et al. (2016). The effect of targeting tolerance of children's negative emotions among anxious parents of children with anxiety disorders: A pilot randomised controlled trial. *Journal of Anxiety Disorders, 42,* 52–59.

Hirshfeld, D. R., Biederman, J., Brody, L., Faraone, S. V., & Rosenbaum, J. F. (1997). Expressed emotion toward children with behavioral inhibition: Associations with maternal anxiety disorder. *Journal of the American Academy of Child and Adolescent Psychiatry, 36,* 910–917.

Hirshfeld-Becker, D. R., Micco, J. A., Simoes, N. A., & Henin, A. (2008). High risk studies and developmental antecedents of anxiety disorders. *American Journal of Medical Genetics Part C: Seminars in Medical Genetics, 148,* 99–117.

Hofmann, S. G., & Smits, J. A. (2008). Cognitive-behavioral therapy for adult anxiety disorders: A meta-analysis of randomized placebo-controlled trials. *Journal of Clinical Psychiatry, 69,* 621–632.

Horvath, A. O., Del Re, A., Flückiger, C., & Symonds, D. (2011). Alliance in individual psychotherapy. *Psychotherapy, 48,* 9–16.

Hudson, J. L., Doyle, A. M., & Gar, N. (2009). Child and maternal influence on parenting behavior in clinically anxious children. *Journal of Clinical Child and Adolescent Psychology, 38,* 256–262.

Hudson, J. L., Keers, R., Roberts, S., Coleman, J. R., Breen, G., Arendt, K., et al. (2015). Clinical predictors of response to cognitive-behavioral therapy in pediatric anxiety disorders: The Genes for Treatment (GxT) Study. *Journal of the American Academy of Child and Adolescent Psychiatry, 54,* 454–463.

Hudson, J. L., Lester, K. J., Lewis, C. M., Tropeano, M., Creswell, C., Collier, D. A., et al. (2013). Predicting outcomes following cognitive behaviour therapy in child anxiety disorders: The influence of genetic, demographic and clinical information. *Journal of Child Psychology and Psychiatry, 54,* 1086–1094.

Hudson, J. L., & Rapee, R. M. (2004). From anxious temperament to disorder: An etiological model. In R. G. Heimberg, C. L. Turk, & D. S. Mennin (Eds.), *Generalized anxiety disorder: Advances in research and practice* (pp. 51–74). New York: Guilford Press.

Ingul, J. M., & Nordahl, H. M. (2013). Anxiety as a risk factor for school absenteeism: What differentiates anxious school attenders from non-attenders? *Annals of General Psychiatry, 12,* 1–9.

James, A. A., Soler, A., & Weatherall, R. R. (2005). Cognitive behavioural therapy for anxiety disorders in children and adolescents. *Cochrane Database System Review, 19*(4): CD004690.

James, A. C., James, G., Cowdrey, F. A., Soler, A., & Choke, A. (2013). Cognitive behavioural therapy for anxiety disorders in children and adolescents. *Cochrane Database System Review, 6:* CD004690.pub4.

Jensen, P. S., Rubio-Stipec, M., Canino, G., Bird, H. R., Dulcan, M. K., Schwab-Stone, M. E., et al. (1999). Parent and child contributions to diagnosis of mental disorder: Are both informants always necessary? *Journal of the American Academy of Child and Adolescent Psychiatry, 38,* 1569–1579.

Kant, G. L., D'Zurilla, T. J., & Maydeu-Olivares, A. (1997). Social problem solving as a mediator of stress-related depression and anxiety in middle-aged and elderly community residents. *Cognitive Therapy and Research, 21,* 73–96.

Kearney, C. A., & Albano, A. M. (2004). The functional profiles of school refusal behavior diagnostic aspects. *Behavior Modification, 28,* 147–161.

Kearney, C. A., & Silverman, W. K. (1996). The evolution and reconciliation of taxonomic strategies for school refusal behavior. *Clinical Psychology: Science and Practice, 3,* 339–354.

Kendall, P. C. (1994). Treating anxiety disorders in children: Results of a randomized clinical trial. *Journal of Consulting and Clinical Psychology, 62,* 100–110.

Kendall, P. C. (2012). Anxiety disorders in youth. In P. C. Kendall (Ed.), *Child and adolescent therapy: Cognitive-behavioral procedures* (4th ed., pp. 143–189). New York: Guilford Press.

Kendall, P. C., Aschenbrand, S. G., & Hudson, J. L. (2003). Child-focused treatment of anxiety. In J. R. Weisz & A. E. Kazdin (Eds.), *Evidence-based psychotherapies for children and adolescents* (pp. 81–100). New York: Guilford Press.

Kendall, P. C., Cummings, C., Villabø, M., Narayanan, M., Treadwell, K., Birmaher, B., et al. (2016). Mediators of change in the Child/Adolescent Anxiety Multimodal Treatment Study. *Journal of Consulting and Clinical Psychology, 84,* 1–14.

Kendall, P. C., Flannery-Schroeder, E., Panichelli-Mindel, S. M., Southam-Gerow, M., Henin, A., & Warman, M. (1997). Therapy for youths with anxiety disorders: A second randomized clincal trial. *Journal of Consulting and Clinical Psychology, 65,* 366–380.

Kendall, P. C., & Hedtke, K. A. (2006). *Cognitive-behavioral therapy for anxious children: Therapist manual.* Ardmore, PA: Workbook.

Kendall, P. C., Hudson, J. L., Gosch, E., Flannery-Schroeder, E., & Suveg, C. (2008). Cognitive-behavioral therapy for anxiety disordered youth: A randomized clinical trial evaluating child and family modalities. *Journal of Consulting and Clinical Psychology, 76,* 282–297.

Kendall, P. C., Kortlander, E., Chansky, T. E., & Brady, E. U. (1992). Comorbidity of anxiety and depression in youth: Treatment implications. *Journal of Consulting And Clinical Psychology, 60,* 869–880.

Kendall, P. C., & Ollendick, T. H. (2005). Setting the research and practice agenda for anxiety in children and adolescence: A topic comes of age. *Cognitive and Behavioral Practice, 11,* 65–74.

Kendall, P. C., Safford, S., Flannery-Schroeder, E., & Webb, A. (2004). Child anxiety treatment: Outcomes in adolescence and impact on substance use and depression at 7.4-year follow-up. *Journal of Consulting and Clinical Psychology, 72,* 276–287.

Kendall, P. C., & Treadwell, K. R. (2007). The role of self-statements as a mediator in treatment for youth with anxiety disorders. *Journal of Consulting and Clinical Psychology, 75,* 380–389.

Kessler, R. C., Berglund, P., Demler, O., Jin, R., Merikangas, K. R., & Walters,

E. E. (2005). Lifetime prevalence and age-of-onset distributions of DSM-IV disorders in the National Comorbidity Survey Replication. *Archives of General Psychiatry, 62*(6), 593–602.

Kessler, R. C., Davis, C. G., & Kendler, K. S. (1997). Childhood adversity and adult psychiatric disorder in the U.S. National Comorbidity Survey. *Psychological Medicine, 27*, 1101–1119.

King, N. J., Ollendick, T. H., & Tonge, B. J. (1995). *School refusal: Assessment and treatment.* Boston: Allyn & Bacon.

King, N. J., Tonge, B. J., Heyne, D., Pritchard, M., Rollings, S., Young, D., et al. (1998). Cognitive-behavioral treatment of school-refusing children: A controlled evaluation. *Journal of the American Academy of Child and Adolescent Psychiatry, 37*, 395–403.

Kortlander, E., Kendall, P. C., & Panichelli-Mindel, S. M. (1997). Maternal expectations and attributions about coping in anxious children. *Journal of Anxiety Disorders, 11*, 297–315.

Ladouceur, R., Blais, F., Freeston, M. H., & Dugas, M. J. (1998). Problem solving and problem orientation in generalized anxiety disorder. *Journal of Anxiety Disorders, 12*, 139–152.

Langley, A. K., Bergman, R. L., McCracken, J., & Piacentini, J. C. (2004). Impairment in childhood anxiety disorders: Preliminary examination of the Child Anxiety Impact Scale—Parent Version. *Journal of Child and Adolescent Psychopharmacology, 14*, 105–114.

Langley, A. K., Cohen, J. A., Mannarino, A. P., Jaycox, L. H., Schonlau, M., Scott, M., et al. (2013). Trauma exposure and mental health problems among school children 15 months post-Hurricane Katrina. *Journal of Child and Adolescent Trauma, 6*, 143–156.

Last, C. G., Hansen, C., & Franco, N. (1998). Cognitive-behavioral treatment of school phobia. *Journal of the American Academy of Child and Adolescent Psychiatry, 37*, 404–411.

Laurent, J., & Ettelson, R. (2001). An examination of the tripartite model of anxiety and depression and its application to youth. *Clinical Child and Family Psychology Review, 4*, 209–230.

Layard, R. (2008). Child mental health: Key to a healthier society. Retrieved from *http://cep.lse.ac.uk/pubs/download/ea035.pdf.*

Leotta, C., Carskadon, M., Acebo, C., Seifer, R., & Quinn, B. (1997). Effects of acute sleep restriction on affective response in adolescents: Preliminary results. *Sleep Research, 26*, 201.

Levy, K., Hunt, C., & Heriot, S. (2007). Treating comorbid anxiety and aggression in children. *Journal of the American Academy of Child and Adolescent Psychiatry, 46*, 1111–1118.

Locke, E. A., & Latham, G. P. (2002). Building a practically useful theory of goal setting and task motivation: A 35-year odyssey. *American Psychologist, 57*, 705–717.

Lyneham, H. J., Abbott, M. J., & Rapee, R. M. (2007). Interrater reliability of the

Anxiety Disorders Interview Schedule for DSM-IV: Child and parent version. *Journal of the American Academy of Child and Adolescent Psychiatry, 46,* 731–736.

Lyneham, H. J., & Rapee, R. M. (2006). Evaluation of therapist-supported parent-implemented CBT for anxiety disorders in rural children. *Behaviour Research and Therapy, 44,* 1287–1300.

Lyneham, H. J., Sburlati, E. S., Abbott, M. J., Rapee, R. M., Hudson, J. L., Tolin, D. F., et al. (2013). Psychometric properties of the Child Anxiety Life Interference Scale (CALIS). *Journal of Anxiety Disorders, 27,* 711–719.

Lyneham, H. J., Street, A. K., Abbott, M. J., & Rapee, R. M. (2008). Psychometric properties of the School Anxiety Scale—Teacher Report (SAS-TR). *Journal of Anxiety Disorders, 22,* 292–300.

Manassis, K., Lee, T. C., Bennett, K., Zhao, X. Y., Mendlowitz, S., Duda, S., et al. (2014). Types of parental involvement in CBT with anxious youth: A preliminary meta-analysis. *Journal of Consulting and Clinical Psychology, 82,* 1163–1172.

Manassis, K., Mendlowitz, S. L., Scapillato, D., Avery, D., Fiksenbaum, L., Freire, M., et al. (2002). Group and individual cognitive-behavioral therapy for childhood anxiety disorders: A randomized trial. *Journal of the American Academy of Child and Adolescent Psychiatry, 41,* 1423–1430.

March, J. S. (2012). *Multidimensional Anxiety Scale for Children* (2nd ed.). Toronto, Ontario, Canada: Multi-Health Systems.

Marks, I. M. (1987). *Fears, phobias, and rituals: Panic, anxiety, and their disorders.* New York: Oxford University Press.

Mathews, A., & Mackintosh, B. (2000). Induced emotional interpretation bias and anxiety. *Journal of Abnormal Psychology, 109,* 602–615.

Maynard, B. R., Heyne, D., Brendel, K. E., Bulanda, J. J., Thompson, A. M., & Pigott, T. D. (2015, August 10). Treatment for school refusal among children and adolescents: A systematic review and meta-analysis. *Research on Social Work Practice.* Epub ahead of print.

McLeod, B. D., Weisz, J. R., & Wood, J. J. (2007). Examining the association between parenting and childhood depression: A meta-analysis. *Clinical Psychology Review, 27,* 986–1003.

Merikangas, K. R., Avenevoli, S., Dierker, L., & Grillon, C. (1999). Vulnerability factors among children at risk for anxiety disorders. *Biological Psychiatry, 46,* 1523–1535.

Micco, J. A., Henin, A., Mick, E., Kim, S., Hopkins, C. A., Biederman, J., et al. (2009). Anxiety and depressive disorders in offspring at high risk for anxiety: A meta-analysis. *Journal of Anxiety Disorders, 23,* 1158–1164.

Milosevic, I., & Radomsky, A. S. (2008). Safety behaviour does not necessarily interfere with exposure therapy. *Behaviour Research and Therapy, 46,* 1111–1118.

Monga, S., Rosenbloom, B. N., Tanha, A., Owens, M., & Young, A. (2015).

Comparison of child–parent and parent-only cognitive-behavioral therapy programs for anxious children aged 5 to 7 years: Short-and long-term outcomes. *Journal of the American Academy of Child and Adolescent Psychiatry, 54*(2), 138–146.

Monk, C. S., Nelson, E. E., McClure, E. B., Mogg, K., Bradley, B. P., Leibenluft, E., et al. (2006). Ventrolateral prefrontal cortex activation and attentional bias in response to angry faces in adolescents with generalized anxiety disorder. *American Journal of Psychiatry, 163,* 1091–1097.

Moore, P. S., Whaley, S. E., & Sigman, M. (2004). Interactions between mothers and children: Impacts of maternal and child anxiety. *Journal of Abnormal Psychology, 113,* 471–476.

Muris, P., Merckelbach, H., Ollendick, T., King, N., & Bogie, N. (2002). Three traditional and three new childhood anxiety questionnaires: Their reliability and validity in a normal adolescent sample. *Behaviour Research and Therapy, 40,* 753–772.

Muris, P., Steerneman, P., Merckelbach, H., Holdrinet, I., & Meesters, C. (1998). Comorbid anxiety symptoms in children with pervasive developmental disorders. *Journal of Anxiety Disorders, 12,* 387–393.

Muris, P., van Zwol, L., Huijding, J., & Mayer, B. (2010). "Mom told me scary things about this animal": Parents installing fear beliefs in their children via the verbal information pathway. *Behaviour Research and Therapy, 48,* 341–346.

Murray, L., Creswell, C., & Cooper, P. (2009). The development of anxiety disorders in childhood: An integrative review. *Psychological Medicine, 39,* 1413–1423.

Murray, L., De Rosnay, M., Pearson, J., Bergeron, C., Schofield, E., Royal-Lawson, M., et al. (2008). Intergenerational transmission of social anxiety: The role of social referencing processes in infancy. *Child Development, 79,* 1049–1064.

Murray, L., Pella, J. E., De Pascalis, L., Arteche, A., Pass, L., Percy, R., et al. (2014). Socially anxious mothers' narratives to their children and their relation to child representations and adjustment. *Development and Psychopathology, 26*(4, Pt. 2), 1531–1546.

Nauta, M. H., Scholing, A., Rapee, R. M., Abbott, M., Spence, S. H., & Waters, A. (2004). A parent-report measure of children's anxiety: Psychometric properties and comparison with child-report in a clinic and normal sample. *Behaviour Research and Therapy, 42,* 813–839.

Nelson, K. (1993). The psychological and social origins of autobiographical memory. *Psychological Science, 4,* 7–14.

Nevo, G. A., & Manassis, K. (2009). Outcomes for treated anxious children: A critical review of long-term follow-up studies. *Depression and Anxiety, 26,* 650–660.

Nisbett, R. E., & Wilson, T. D. (1977). Telling more than we can know: Verbal reports on mental processes. *Psychological Review, 84,* 231–259.

Nolen-Hoeksema, S., Girgus, J. S., & Seligman, M. E. (1992). Predictors and consequences of childhood depressive symptoms: A 5-year longitudinal study. *Journal of Abnormal Psychology, 101,* 405–422.

Ollendick, T. H., & Mayer, J. A. (1984). School phobia. In S. M. Turner (Ed.), *Behavioral theories and treatment of anxiety* (pp. 367–411). New York: Springer.

Owens, J. A., Spirito, A., & McGuinn, M. (2001). The Children's Sleep Habits Questionnaire (CSHQ): Psychometric properties of a survey instrument for school-aged children. *Sleep, 23,* 1043–1051.

Owens, J. A., Spirito, A., McGuinn, M., & Nobile, C. (2000). Sleep habits and sleep disturbance in elementary school-aged children. *Journal of Developmental and Behavioral Pediatrics, 21,* 27–36.

Paine, S., & Gradisar, M. (2011). A randomised controlled trial of cognitive-behaviour therapy for behavioural insomnia of childhood in school-aged children. *Behaviour Research and Therapy, 49,* 379–388.

Parker, G. (1983). Parental "affectionless control" as an antecedent to adult depression: A risk factor delineated. *Archives of General Psychiatry, 40,* 956–960.

Parkinson, M., & Creswell, C. (2011). Worry and problem-solving skills and beliefs in primary school children. *British Journal of Clinical Psychology, 50,* 106–112.

Pennant, M. E., Loucas, C. E., Whittington, C., Creswell, C., Fonagy, P., Fuggle, P., et al. (2015). Computerised therapies for anxiety and depression in children and young people: A systematic review and meta-analysis. *Behaviour Research and Therapy, 67,* 1–18.

Peris, T. S., Compton, S. N., Kendall, P. C., Birmaher, B., Sherrill, J., March, J., et al. (2015). Trajectories of change in youth anxiety during cognitive-behavior therapy. *Journal of Consulting and Clinical Psychology, 83,* 239–252.

Polanczyk, G. V., Salum, G. A., Sugaya, L. S., Caye, A., & Rohde, L. A. (2015). Annual research review: A meta-analysis of the worldwide prevalence of mental disorders in children and adolescents. *Journal of Child Psychology and Psychiatry, 56,* 345–365.

Puleo, C. M., & Kendall, P. C. (2011). Anxiety disorders in typically developing youth: Autism spectrum symptoms as a predictor of cognitive-behavioral treatment. *Journal of Autism and Developmental Disorders, 41,* 275–286.

Rachman, S. (1981). Part I: Unwanted intrusive cognitions. *Advances in Behaviour Research and Therapy, 3,* 89–99.

Rapee, R. M. (2000). Group treatment of children with anxiety disorders: Outcome and predictors of treatment response. *Australian Journal of Psychology, 52*(3), 125–129.

Rapee, R. M. (2003). The influence of comorbidity on treatment outcome for children and adolescents with anxiety disorders. *Behaviour Research and Therapy, 41,* 105–112.

Rapee, R. M., Abbott, M. J., & Lyneham, H. J. (2006). Bibliotherapy for children with anxiety disorders using written materials for parents: A randomized controlled trial. *Journal of Consulting and Clinical Psychology, 74,* 436–444.

Rapee, R. M., & Heimberg, R. G. (1997). A cognitive-behavioral model of anxiety in social phobia. *Behaviour Research and Therapy, 35,* 741–756.

Rapee, R. M., & Lim, L. (1992). Discrepancy between self- and observer ratings of performance in social phobics. *Journal of Abnormal Psychology, 101,* 728–731.

Rapee, R. M., Lyneham, H. J., Hudson, J. L., Kangas, M., Wuthrich, V. M., & Schniering, C. A. (2013). Effect of comorbidity on treatment of anxious children and adolescents: Results from a large, combined sample. *Journal of the American Academy of Child and Adolescent Psychiatry, 52,* 47–56.

Rapee, R. M., Lyneham, H. J., Schniering, C. A., Wuthrich, V., Abbott, M. A., Hudson, J. L., et al. (2006). *Cool Kids: Child and adolescent anxiety program.* Sydney, Australia: Centre for Emotional Health, Macquarie University.

Rapee, R. M., & Spence, S. H. (2004). The etiology of social phobia: Empirical evidence and an initial model. *Clinical Psychology Review, 24,* 737–767.

Remmerswaal, D., Muris, P., Mayer, B., & Smeets, G. (2010). "Will a Cuscus bite you, if he shows his teeth?": Inducing a fear-related confirmation bias in children by providing verbal threat information to their mothers. *Journal of Anxiety Disorders, 24,* 540–546.

Research Units on Pediatric Psychopharmacology Anxiety Study Group. (2002). The Pediatric Anxiety Rating Scale (PARS): Development and psychometric properties. *Journal of the American Academy of Child and Adolescent Psychiatry, 41,* 1061–1069.

Reynolds, K. C., & Alfano, C. A. (2016). Things that go bump in the night: Frequency and predictors of nightmares in anxious and nonanxious children. *Behavioral Sleep Medicine, 14,* 442–456.

Reynolds, S., Wilson, C., Austin, J., & Hooper, L. (2012). Effects of psychotherapy for anxiety in children and adolescents: A meta-analytic review. *Clinical Psychology Review, 32,* 251–262.

Roy-Byrne, P. P., Davidson, K. W., Kessler, R. C., Asmundson, G. J., Goodwin, R. D., Kubzansky, L., et al. (2008). Anxiety disorders and comorbid medical illness. *General Hospital Psychiatry, 30,* 208–225.

Rubin, K. H., Burgess, K. B., & Hastings, P. D. (2002). Stability and social-behavioral consequences of toddlers' inhibited temperament and parenting behaviors. *Child Development, 73*(2), 483–495.

Rutter, M., Bailey, A., & Lord, C. (2003). *The Social Communication Questionnaire (SCQ).* Los Angeles: Western Psychological Services.

Rynn, M. A., Walkup, J. T., Compton, S. N., Sakolsky, D. J., Sherrill, J. T., Shen, S., et al. (2015), Child/adolescent anxiety multimodal study: Evaluating safety. *Journal of the American Academy of Child and Adolescent Psychiatry, 54*(3), 180–190.

Safran, J. D., & Wallner, L. K. (1991). The relative predictive validity of two therapeutic alliance measures in cognitive therapy. *Psychological Assessment: A Journal of Consulting and Clinical Psychology, 3,* 188–195.

Salkovskis, P. M. (1991). The importance of behaviour in the maintenance of anxiety and panic: A cognitive account. *Behavioural Psychotherapy, 19,* 6–19.

Salum, G., Mogg, K., Bradley, B., Gadelha, A., Pan, P., Tamanaha, A., et al.

(2013). Threat bias in attention orienting: Evidence of specificity in a large community-based study. *Psychological Medicine, 43,* 733–745.

Schlarb, A. A., Velten-Schurian, K., Poets, C. F., & Hautzinger, M. (2011). First effects of a multicomponent treatment for sleep disorders in children. *Nature and Science of Sleep, 3,* 1.

Schleider, J. L., Patel, A., Krumholz, L., Chorpita, B. F., & Weisz, J. R. (2015). Relation between parent symptomatology and youth problems: Multiple mediation through family income and parent–youth stress. *Child Psychiatry and Human Development, 46,* 1–9.

Silverman, W. K., & Albano, A. M. (1996). *Anxiety Disorders Interview Schedule for DSM-IV and Parent Interview Schedule.* New York: Oxford University Press.

Silverman, W. K., Kurtines, W. M., Jaccard, J., & Pina, A. A. (2009). Directionality of change in youth anxiety treatment involving parents: An initial examination. *Journal of Consulting and Clinical Psychology, 77,* 474–485.

Silverman, W. K., & Nelles, W. B. (1988). The Anxiety Disorders Interview Schedule for children. *Journal of the American Academy of Child and Adolescent Psychiatry, 27,* 772–778.

Silverman, W. K., Saavedra, L. M., & Pina, A. A. (2001). Test–retest reliability of anxiety symptoms and diagnoses with the Anxiety Disorders Interview Schedule for DSM-IV: Child And Parent Versions. *Journal of the American Academy of Child and Adolescent Psychiatry, 40,* 937–944.

Simon, E., van der Sluis, C., Muris, P., Thompson, E., & Cartwright-Hatton, S. (2014). Anxiety in preadolescent children: What happens if we don't treat it, and what happens if we do? *Psychopathology Review, 1,* 28–50.

Spence, S. H. (1995). *Social skills training: Enhancing social competence with children and adolescents.* Windsor, UK: NFER-Nelson.

Spence, S. H. (1998). A measure of anxiety symptoms among children. *Behaviour Research and Therapy, 36,* 545–566.

Spence, S. H., Donovan, C., & Brechman-Toussaint, M. (1999). Social skills, social outcomes, and cognitive features of childhood social phobia. *Journal of Abnormal Psychology, 108,* 211–221.

Spence, S. H., Donovan, C., & Brechman-Toussaint, M. (2000). The treatment of childhood social phobia: The effectiveness of a social skills training-based, cognitive-behavioural intervention, with and without parental involvement. *Journal of Child Psychology and Psychiatry, 41,* 713–726.

Spence, S. H., Rapee, R., McDonald, C., & Ingram, M. (2001). The structure of anxiety symptoms among preschoolers. *Behaviour Research and Therapy, 39,* 1293–1316.

Stallard, P. (2003). *Think Good—Feel Good: A cognitive behaviour therapy workbook for children and young people.* Chichester, UK: Wiley.

Stallard, P. (2005). *A clinician's guide to Think Good—Feel Good: Using CBT with children and young people.* Chichester, UK: Wiley.

Stallard, P., Simpson, N., Anderson, S., Hibbert, S., & Osborn, C. (2007). The

FRIENDS emotional health programme: Initial findings from a school-based project. *Child and Adolescent Mental Health, 12,* 32–37.

Stallard, P., Udwin, O., Goddard, M., & Hibbert, S. (2007). The availability of cognitive behaviour therapy within specialist child and adolescent mental health services (CAMHS): A national survey. *Behavioural and Cognitive Psychotherapy, 35,* 501–505.

Steketee, G., Frost, R., & Bogart, K. (1996). The Yale–Brown Obsessive Compulsive Scale: Interview versus self-report. *Behaviour Research and Therapy, 34,* 675–684.

Stopa, L., & Clark, D. M. (1993). Cognitive processes in social phobia. *Behaviour Research and Therapy, 31,* 255–267.

Storch, E. A., Murphy, T. K., Lack, C. W., Geffken, G. R., Jacob, M. L., & Goodman, W. K. (2008). Sleep-related problems in pediatric obsessive–compulsive disorder. *Journal of Anxiety Disorders, 22,* 877–885.

Taboas, W. R., McKay, D., Whiteside, S. P., & Storch, E. A. (2015). Parental involvement in youth anxiety treatment: Conceptual bases, controversies, and recommendations for intervention. *Journal of Anxiety Disorders, 30,* 16–18.

Teasdale, J. D. (1988). Cognitive vulnerability to persistent depression. *Cognition and Emotion, 2,* 247–274.

Thirlwall, K., Cooper, P., & Creswell, C. (2016). *Guided parent-delivered cognitive behavioral therapy for childhood anxiety: Predictors of treatment response.* Manuscript under review.

Thirlwall, K., Cooper, P. J., Karalus, J., Voysey, M., Willetts, L., & Creswell, C. (2013). Treatment of child anxiety disorders via guided parent-delivered cognitive-behavioural therapy: Randomised controlled trial. *British Journal of Psychiatry, 203,* 436–444.

Thirlwall, K., & Creswell, C. (2010). The impact of maternal control on children's anxious cognitions, behaviours and affect: An experimental study. *Behaviour Research and Therapy, 48,* 1041–1046.

Thompson, S., & Rapee, R. M. (2002). The effect of situational structure on the social performance of socially anxious and non-anxious participants. *Journal of Behavior Therapy and Experimental Psychiatry, 33,* 91–102.

Tiwari, S., Kendall, P. C., Hoff, A. L., Harrison, J. P., & Fizur, P. (2013). Characteristics of exposure sessions as predictors of treatment response in anxious youth. *Journal of Clinical Child and Adolescent Psychology, 42,* 34–43.

Waite, P., Codd, J., & Creswell, C. (2015). Interpretation of ambiguity: Differences between children and adolescents with and without an anxiety disorder. *Journal of Affective Disorders, 188,* 194–201.

Waite, P., & Creswell, C. (2014). Children and adolescents referred for treatment of anxiety disorders: Differences in clinical characteristics. *Journal of Affective Disorders, 167,* 326–332.

Walter, D., Hautmann, C., Rizk, S., Petermann, M., Minkus, J., Sinzig, J., et al. (2010). Short term effects of inpatient cognitive behavioral treatment of adolescents with anxious–depressed school absenteeism: An observational study. *European Child and Adolescent Psychiatry, 19,* 835–844.

Waters, A. M., Craske, M. G., Bergman, R. L., & Treanor, M. (2008). Threat interpretation bias as a vulnerability factor in childhood anxiety disorders. *Behaviour Research and Therapy, 46,* 39–47.

Waters, A. M., Ford, L. A., Wharton, T. A., & Cobham, V. E. (2009). Cognitive-behavioural therapy for young children with anxiety disorders: Comparison of a child + parent condition versus a parent only condition. *Behaviour Research and Therapy, 47,* 654–662.

Waters, A. M., Wharton, T. A., Zimmer-Gembeck, M. J., & Craske, M. G. (2008). Threat-based cognitive biases in anxious children: Comparison with non-anxious children before and after cognitive behavioural treatment. *Behaviour Research and Therapy, 46,* 358–374.

Weems, C. F., Silverman, W. K., Rapee, R. M., & Pina, A. A. (2003). The role of control in childhood anxiety disorders. *Cognitive Therapy and Research, 27,* 557–568.

Wheatcroft, R., & Creswell, C. (2007). Parents' cognitions and expectations about their pre-school children: The contribution of parental anxiety and child anxiety. *British Journal of Developmental Psychology, 25,* 435–441.

Wilson, C., & Hughes, C. (2011). Worry, beliefs about worry and problem solving in young children. *Behavioural and Cognitive Psychotherapy, 39,* 507–521.

Wood, J. J., Drahota, A., Sze, K., Har, K., Chiu, A., & Langer, D. A. (2009). Cognitive behavioral therapy for anxiety in children with autism spectrum disorders: A randomized, controlled trial. *Journal of Child Psychology and Psychiatry, 50,* 224–234.

Wood, J. J., Ehrenreich-May, J., Alessandri, M., Fujii, C., Renno, P., Laugeson, E., et al. (2015). Cognitive behavioral therapy for early adolescents with autism spectrum disorders and clinical anxiety: A randomized, controlled trial. *Behavior Therapy, 46,* 7–19.

Wood, J. J., McLeod, B. D., Sigman, M., Hwang, W. C., & Chu, B. C. (2003). Parenting and childhood anxiety: Theory, empirical findings, and future directions. *Journal of Child Psychology and Psychiatry, 44,* 134–151.

Index

Note. f or t following a page number indicates a figure or a table.